God Still Works Miracles:

A Journal of One Couple's Struggle with Guillain-Barre' Syndrome

By
Romayne & Bob Harkcom

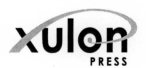

God Still Works Miracles: A Journal of One Couple's Struggle with Guillain-Barre' Syndrome
by Romayne & Bob Harkcom

Printed in the United States of America

ISBN 9781615795369

Unless otherwise indicated, Bible quotations are taken from The New Revised Standard Version of the Bible. Copyright © 1989 by World Bible Publishers, Inc.

www.xulonpress.com

W e would like to take this opportunity to thank Sarah Reiber and Michelle Levigne for their assistance in helping us get this book ready for publishing and for directing us to Xulon Press to have it published.

Foreword

Dear friends:

Ijust wanted to let you know about my experience with Guillain-Barre' Syndrome. In June of 2005, I contracted bronchitis. After taking medications for the bronchitis, I began to recover from that. Then in July of 2005, I started getting tingling in my hands and feet. Then after another day or two, I was down and out of it. My husband took me to the emergency room and they couldn't find anything wrong. They sent me home with pain medicine.

A week later, I continued to get worse, so I went back to the emergency room in an ambulance. After many extensive tests, they finally called a neurological doctor, who advised them to do a spinal tap, which showed the high protein levels, and then I was diagnosed with Guillain-Barre' Syndrome.

We were scared to death when they told my husband and me what I had. We had never heard of it, and no one else knew anything about it either. They had to life-flight me to another hospital that had better facilities. By the time this all happened, I was completely paralyzed and could barely move my head.

I was in the hospital and rehabilitation center for eight months. When I was released to go home, I went to another rehabilitation center three times a week for another nine months. I am still working out at a gym and at home.

At the present time, "THANKS BE TO GOD," I am able to walk with a cane in the house and walk outside with help. I'm hoping with the help of God that I will continue to improve. The support of my husband, family and Christian friends has helped me tremendously with the battle of Guillain-Barre' Syndrome.

I would be willing to talk to anyone who would have any questions about their fears of Guillain-Barre' Syndrome. My phone number is 814-267-4545. Please leave a message and phone number if I'm not at home at the time you call.

Sincerely yours,

Romayne Harkcom
Berlin. PA

God Still Works Miracles

Note:

I wrote this as a speech that I was going to give to our congregation in our church, but because we were going to Florida, and Pastor could not fit my speech into any of the services, when we came back from Florida he never mentioned it, so I never gave the speech.

I'm here today to tell the story of God's love and how He worked a miracle in my life. God laid it on my heart to give this testimony. Pastor John asked me about a year ago to give the testimony of my problem with GBS (Guillain-Barre' Syndrome). I've never had the courage to talk in front of a group of people in my life, so I'm very nervous, but with God's help I'll be able to tell you my story. It all began about three years ago. I thought I was in pretty good health. I went to Curves about five or six times a week. Bob and I walked about two miles on a regular basis. We went line dancing often and were active in other things. Then in June 2005, I came down with a bad cough and was pretty sick for about two weeks and finally went to the doctor. He diagnosed me with bronchitis and started me on some antibiotics. I was finally starting to feel better and thought I was over it, when I woke up with a bad pain in my back, and my feet and hands were tingling. I didn't think much about it and thought it would go away, but it continued to get worse.

We got up Sunday and started getting ready for church, but things were not going very well. So Bob insisted we go to the emergency room. I was there all day. They did all kind of tests and couldn't find anything wrong. They sent me home with pain pills and scheduled me for an MRI on Monday and to go to therapy at the Commons on Tuesday. When we got home from the emergency room, I was worse then ever. Bob called the emergency room and told them that I was worse and the pills were not helping. They said there wasn't anything else they could do. They ran all the tests there were. I would have to wait until Monday and call the family doctor.

We did that, and all they did was prescribe stronger medicine. This did not help at all. I followed their instructions and went for the MRI on Monday and for therapy on Tuesday. The therapist said he didn't know what to do for me, so he just put a heating pad on my back. That eased the pain, but didn't take the tingling or numbness away. We discovered later on why the heating pad helped relieve the pain. The doctor said it was because I had pneumonia. That's what caused the pain in my back. When we left therapy that day, they had to loan me a walker and it took Bob and the therapist to get me to the car. I had a pretty hard time getting into the house, but I made it.

I was going to the bathroom on Tuesday, and on the way back to the living room. I fell. It seemed strange that I didn't hurt myself. It was because the nerves were going. The pain was coming later. I managed to get myself back on my feet.

On Wednesday, Nancy Schrock brought some soup over for us. At that time, I couldn't stand up by myself. Bob and Nancy tried to get me up, but couldn't. They decided to call 911. By this time I was pretty well out of it. As they were taking me to the emergency room, Bob was following the ambulance and prayed that there would be someone at the emergency room who could diagnose the problem. When we arrived, there was a doctor on duty, and after looking at the test results and symptoms he called a neurologist, who advised him to do a spinal tap to determine the protein level. The test came back positive and they diagnosed me with having Guillain-Barre' Syndrome.

They admitted me to ICU. While they were getting me into bed, I had two seizures. They got me calmed and medicated and I rested that night. I think the seizures might have caused me to have problems with my memory. From this point on, I don't remember much of what happened for the next two months.

Thursday morning, July 24th, a doctor from Westmoreland Hospital came in to run tests. At 5:00pm that day, the doctor called Bob in and confirmed a severe case of Guillain-Barre' Syndrome, and didn't give us much hope. She explained GBS was a virus that attacks the peripheral nerves and destroys them. I needed to be life-flighted to Westmoreland Hospital immediately. I don't remember the helicopter ride.

During my stay at the hospital, I had many visitors, especially Pastor John, who came at least every week. He gave me communion and prayed for me. I got a lot of cards, which was great. This let me know that everyone was thinking about me.

Also during my time in ICU, I saw many miracles, but the greatest miracle came when my heart stopped working properly. After many prayers from family, friends, church family and many other churches, even some as far away as Texas, it was healed. The heart doctor didn't give me much hope, but we continued to pray. The second week, my heart started to respond and to improve. The heart doctor ran another test and said it showed the heart perfectly normal. He couldn't explain why. We told him it was all the prayers and God did the healing. He said he agreed, because there was no medical reason why the heart would come back like that. Now that the heart was functioning properly, they could continue the treatment on the GBS.

At this point of time, I had lost control of my hands, arms, legs and everything except the limited ability to still move my head. Even my speech was affected, and I had to do some exercises to help me swallow. The doctor said we had a long road ahead of us. He couldn't tell us how much I would improve, because everyone's reaction to GBS is different.

I remember when Bob would come in the morning, I would tell him to please help me get out of this bed. After a couple times of me asking him this, he said, "Okay. If you sit up, I will help you get up." I think this was the first time I realized how sick I really was, because I couldn't even lift my arms, let alone try to sit up.

As time went on, with many prayers and help and support from so many people too numerous to mention, I finally progressed, with many setbacks, to where I am today.

I had a lot of urinary tract infections and numerous blocked bowels and an infected eye, which left me with scar tissue and bad vision in that eye. I had internal bleeding due to taking blood thinners. They gave me seven units of blood. And I had a lot of other problems.

At this time, they began therapy on me. They started off just two times a day, working my fingers, my arms, my legs and feet. In between the times they would do it, Bob would exercise me. Then they tried to stand me up by using what they called a standing tilt table. It took four people to get me on it. Then I could only stand about thirty seconds. After a number of times, I could stand two minutes. As I continued to improve, they moved me to Westmoreland Rehab Center for more aggressive therapy.

One of the many things they did there was set me in a jerry chair. I could sit up for about ten minutes at first. After a while, they put me in a wheelchair. I couldn't stand the pain, but I knew with the Lord's help, I had to do this if I wanted to get better. One of the hardest things I had to do was when they tried to stand me up. They would have three people do it. one on each arm, and one would wrap a sheet around me and pull me up while standing between the parallel bars. I could only stand about ten seconds at first. I progressed to five minutes.

I was released from the hospital in December to go to The Patriot in Somerset. When I arrived there, I couldn't sit up myself and couldn't move my legs. With dedication and hard work, and with Bob pushing me, we started seeing some improvement.

On December 10th, Diane Pechinski, who is a faith healer along with Pastor John and some members of the church, came to The Patriot to pray for me. We joined hands in a prayer circle and she prayed. After the prayer, she talked with me privately and it seemed that from that time on, I improved more rapidly. This wasn't an instant cure, but it was another miracle.

By this time, I had most of my senses back and knew what was going on. I was suffering a lot of pain and it was really hard for me to do the exercises and the therapy. God would not let me give up. I knew I had to continue on, pain or not. The pain was so bad that when Bob kissed me or held my hand, I couldn't stand it very long.

The therapists at The Patriot were wonderful. They were caring but demanding, and pushed me to the limit. They did everything they could to help me. The worse thing I can remember trying to do was to stand up in what they called a standing frame. I called it a box. It would take three people to get me up into it. They would push a board behind me and let me stand as long as I could, which wasn't very long. As I improved, they started me walking with a walker, two people holding my arms and one holding my knees, so they wouldn't buckle. This was very difficult. I continued to work hard every day and I progressed to the point where I could go home with a walker and a wheelchair, in the middle of February 2006.

We could not have made it through without the support of God, church family, friends and relatives, with all the cards, donations, food, visitors and people who came to the house to help with continued therapy. We are still going to the gym three times a week for therapy. I thank God that I can continue to do this, and for His continued healing in my life.

Through this trial, both of us have a closer relationship with God through Christ and with each other. I realize we cannot stop trials, so instead I try to get as much good from them as I can, and I now see my trials as faithful friends that point me to God and conform me into His image. As we read in the book of James, chapter one, verses 2 to 4, "Count it all joy, my brethren, when you meet various trials, for you know the testing of your faith produces steadfastness. And let steadfastness have its full effect, that you may be perfect and complete, lacking in nothing."

Through all this, I've come to realize that there is nothing as important in this life as the promise and the guarantee that comes to us through our faith in Jesus Christ that we will have eternal life with Him someday.

I thank and praise the Lord every day for His blessings. I hope that through this experience, I have been able to witness to others the love of Christ.

I just want to say one more thing. Through all this experience with GBS, my husband, Bob, has been so supportive of me. He never missed a day to be with me the seven months I was in the hospital and The Patriot. He was so wonderful and helpful to me. If he wouldn't have been there, I don't know what would have happened to me.

When I was leaving The Patriot, the therapists gave me a surprise going home party. And when I arrived at my home the next day, our friends had a welcome home party for me, another surprise. What wonderful friends we have.

Everyone has been so wonderful to me. I just want to thank all of you for your support.

Romayne & Bob Harkcom

God makes His promises to everyone through His Holy Word. He reveals His healing powers and love if we would totally put our hope and trust in Him, we will find him in our bodies and souls.

There are many references to healing in the Bible. Some that give us strength are found in the following verses from the New Revised Standard Version (copyright 1989):

Malachi 4:2
But for you who revere my name, the son of righteousness shall rise with healing in its wings

Matthew 4:23
Jesus went throughout Galilee teaching in their synagogues and proclaiming the good news of the kingdom and curing every disease and every sickness among the people.

Psalm 30:1-5
1 I will extol you, O Lord, for you have drawn me up, and did not let my foes rejoice over me. 2 O Lord my God, I cried to you for help, and you have healed me. 3 O Lord, you brought up my soul from Sheol, restored me to life from among those gone

down to the pit. 4 Sing praises to the Lord, O you his faithful ones, and give thanks to his holy name. 5 For his anger is but for a moment; his favor is for a lifetime. Weeping may linger for the night, but joy comes with the morning.

Psalm 103:1-6

1 Bless the Lord, O my soul, and all that is within me, bless his holy name. 2 Bless the Lord, O my soul, and do not forget all his benefits – 3 who forgives all your iniquity, who heals all your diseases, 4 who redeems your life from the pit, who crowns you with steadfast love and mercy, 5 who satisfies you with good as long as you live, so that your youth is renewed like the eagle's. 6 The Lord works vindication and justice for all who are oppressed.

Acts 10: 34-43

34 Then Peter began to speak to them: I truly understand that God shows no partiality, 35 but in every nation anyone who fears him and does what is right is acceptable to him. 36 You know the message you sent to the people of Israel, preaching peace by Jesus Christ – he is Lord of all. 37 That message spread throughout Judea, beginning in Galilee after the baptism John announced: 38 how God anointed Jesus of Nazareth with the Holy Spirit and with power; how he went about doing good and healing all who were oppressed by the devil, for God was with him. 39 We are witnesses to all that he did both in Judea and in Jerusalem. They put him to death by hanging him on a tree; 40 but God raised him on the third day and allowed him to appear, 41 not to

all the people but to us who were chosen by God as witnesses, and who ate and drank with him after he rose from the dead. 42 He commanded us to preach to the people and to testify that he is the one ordained by God as judge of the living and the dead. 43 All the prophets testify about him that everyone who believes in him receives forgiveness of sins through his name.

DEFINITION OF GBS

Guillain-Barre' Syndrome is an autoimmune disorder which causes inflammation of the peripheral nerves.

GBS usually involves loss of the nerve's myelin sheath, which slows the conduction of impulses through the nerve.

GBS may also cause destruction of the axon of the nerve cell, which blocks conduction through the nerve.

The syndrome results in muscle weakness, paralysis, and / or sensory disturbances.

Symptoms can be compared to these of polio.

GBS damages the nerves that affect the arms, legs, lungs, throat, heart, and / or eyes.

Symptoms and signs of GBS can vary greatly among patients.

GBS affects about one to two in every 100,000 people per year, making it the most common cause of rapidly acquired paralysis in the U.S.

Some patients require assisted breathing if muscles in the chest are affected.

The syndrome is extremely painful. During paralysis, the pain stems from muscles being paralyzed, as well as lying positions because of the inability to move and because of the nerves not being able to send signals to the muscles.

Later in the progression of GBS, pain stems from the feeling of nerves coming back to life. The pain is knife like and burning, and the patient can also have hypersensitivity to touch. Even their own clothes or bed linens can feel like knives against the skin. During this time patients must also begin physical therapy so that they can heal faster, and this causes great pain as well.

The symptoms are usually temporary, but can be recurring.

Relapses occur in about 3% of patients.

Death can occur in about 4% of cases, about 80% recover completely, 5-10% are permanently severely disabled.

Although recovered, patients can sometimes feel tingling and numbness in fingers and toes and have problems fully using their hands.

The cause of GBS is unknown, but the onset of the syndrome usually occurs shortly after a microbial infection, minor surgery, vaccinations, or childbirth.

There is no known cause or cure for GBS, but there are treatments to lessen symptoms.

There are many names for GBS including: Landry's paralysis, Kussmaul-Landry syndrome, Guillain-Barre'-Strohl syndrome, acute ascending polyradiculoneuritie, acute inflammatory demyelinating polyradiculoneuropathy, celluroradiculoneuritis, and schwannosis.

Idiopathic means that the cause of the disease is unknown. Acute means that it is rapid. Inflammatory means that it is irritating. Demyelinating means that myelin is destroyed.

May 1st is International GBS Awareness Day.

TREATMENT

There is no cure for Guillain-Barre' syndrome, but symptoms can be treated

The syndrome causes extreme pain, especially while the nerves heal, so patients need medication and special care to reduce pain. Patients also need special care to avoid problems associated with long periods of lying in bed, such as bedsores, blood clots, and pneumonia.

If GBS affects the chest muscles, patients will need a ventilator to breathe for them. If the patient requires a ventilator for more than two weeks, a tracheotomy is performed, and instead of a pipe being inserted into the nose or mouth, the tube is placed through a small slit in the patient's throat and directly into the windpipe.

Immune-therapy targets the patient's antibodies. This therapy reduces the damage to the patient's tissue, and shortens the duration of the disease. GBS is thought to be an autoimmune disorder, which causes a patient's immune system to attack the patient's own body.

Plasmapheresis, or plasma exchange (PE), takes the antibodies from a patient's blood to prevent them from attacking the body. The body continuously produces antibodies, so the patient must continue to undergo PE each time the body produces enough antibodies for the attack to resume. Patients must continue plasma therapy until they begin to recover.

During PE, a patient is connected to a machine that slowly removes blood and takes out antibodies. The method can be compared to dialysis. Red and white blood cells are separated from the diseased plasma, and is replaced by fresh donated plasma. There are various ways to do this, including taking out and replacing plasma using a large syringe. Some hospitals place a catheter into a large artery, leaving the two ends outside the body. The ends are then connected to a dialysis machine and the old and new antibodies are exchanged. The catheter remains in the patient between treatments.

Intravenous immunoglobulin infusion, or IVIg, works in much the same way that plasmapheresis does. High doses of donor antibodies are injected into the patient's blood. The donor antibodies outnumber the patient's own infected antibodies and slow down the disease. The white blood cells that produce the unwanted antibodies are also slowed. Treatment can vary depending on the hospital, just as with PE. Usually plasma is dissolved in a liquid and administered through an IV in the person's wrist.

Immunadsorption (Imad) is much like PE. A catheter is inserted and immunoglobulins are removed, but in PE immunoglobulins and plasma are discarded. The blood is treated by two machines to separate antibodies and plasma.

Before these treatments, patients simply healed on their own, and recovery took much longer. Before ventilators, patients died of suffocation.

Neurologists, scientists, immunologists, and pharmacologists are working to prevent GBS and find better treatments, and possibly a cure. Research is being done on the immune system to discover the reason behind the syndrome. Other discoveries are being made about the nervous system and how attacks begin and end. Still others study how viruses affect GBS.

HISTORY

Early19th century-medical papers begin showing descriptions of progressive numbness and weakness followed by spontaneous recovery, the symptoms of GBS

1859- The best description of acute ascending paralysis was written by the French Jean Baptiste Octave Landry de The'zillat, who described 10 cases of GBS-like symptoms.

1892- Ostler categorized six classes of polyneuropathy, with one category, acute febrile polyneuritis, closely relating to what is now known as Guillain-Barre' syndrome.

1916- George Guillain, Jean Alexandre Barre' and Andre Strohl discovered the key diagnostic abnormality of increased spinal fluid protein production, but normal cell count.

1920- Guillain and Barre' publish *Travaux neurologiques de Guerre,* in which they distinguish GBS from Landry's paralysis and nerve gas poisoning.

Late 1940s- Respiratory ICUs and use of positive pressure ventilation reduces GBS deaths.

1969- Scientists show the connection between GBS and lymphocytic infiltration in spinal roots and nerves.

1976- Hoping to avoid an epidemic, Swine Flu vaccination was given to 50 million people in 10 weeks, setting an immunization world record. However, at the same time many of those who were vaccinated acquired Guillain-Barre' syndrome.

1978- Use of the plasma exchange first reported in GBS patients.

1981- GBS symposium updates GBS research, especially its immune and pathologic features.

DIAGNOSIS OF GBS

A thorough examination is required for a patient to be diagnosed with Guillain-Barre' syndrome.

A physician will determine if the symptoms occur equally on both sides of the body, check for increasing weakness, look for loss of tendon reflexes and check for signs of a previous infection.

Laboratory tests will likely also be included, such as blood and urine tests, stool tests, x-rays, scans, Lumbar puncture, Nerve Condition Velocity test (NCV), nerve biopsy, MRI, or electromyogram (EMG).

A lumbar puncture examines a person's spinal fluid. It's also known as a spinal tap. For GBS, the spinal fluid will be normal except for a rise in the protein level in the cerebrospinal fluid.

A Nerve Condition Velocity test examines how well nerves function. If a nerve has damaged myelin transmit signals, they will transmit slower than healthy ones, and nerves with destroyed axons cannot transmit at all. During the test, flat electrodes are put on the person's skin above the nerves to be tested. Different electrodes emit different levels of electrical impulse through the nerve. The time the nerve takes to respond is calculated and doctors calculate whether or not the nerves are damaged or destroyed.

An electromyogram is used to determine whether a patient has a muscle disorder, or if they have muscle weakness due to a neurological disorder such as GBS. During the test, a nerve is stimulated and the muscle activity is measured. An electrode is pushed into the muscle to be tested and connected to a monitor. The measurements of muscle fiber movement are shown on the screen.

Magnetic Resonance Imaging gives doctors images of one's internal body. It uses strong magnets and a radio antenna to send and receive pictures of the body. For GBS patients, an MRI is used to look at the brain, spinal cord, and nerves to determine damage.

A nerve biopsy may be required in rare cases. A small section of a nerve is removed and examined under a microscope for any sign of damage.

Romayne's Story Begins

I was born and raised on a farm in western Pennsylvania. There were eight children, including me: six boys and two girls. Our family worked hard on the farm. Since I was a girl and one of the youngest, I didn't have to do much of the barn work. My chores were washing the milkers and feeding the chickens. Housework was more up my alley; although my mom was a wonderful cook, I didn't learn how to cook until I got married and moved out to our own apartment.

When I was a baby, just crawling I fell into a spring which was the water supply for the house. I don't know how long I was in the water, but my sister found me and pulled me out and saved my life.

When I was nine years old my brother and I were playing outside when a rare tornado came through our farm. My mother and sister got us in the house just in time. The tornado blew down all the big pine trees around the house, but by the grace of God, none of them fell on the house. It also blew the end of the barn out, knocked over the corn crib, and caused many other damages. The strange thing about this was that our farm was the only one that had any damages.

I remember many people coming to see all the damage because no one else in the area received any damages.

Mom took us to church and Sunday school. We got all dressed up on Sunday mornings, and away we went. When I turned 12, I was baptized and the Lord worked in me - I was changing. One day a minister came to our house, and my brother and I renewed our commitment to Christ.

I was married to my husband, Bob, while still in school. After I graduated from high school, we lived with my parents for about a year; Bob worked for my dad at that time. Bob took a job at a factory, and we moved into our own apartment. By this time, our son was about a year old.

The economy started to go bad, and Bob lost his job. I had an aunt and uncle who lived near Cleveland, Ohio, who had told Bob that anytime he wanted, he could come stay with them and look for work. We finally decided that this was what we should do.

In 1960, Bob left for Ohio and our son, Bob Jr., and I moved back in with my parents. My husband got a job the second week he was there, in a factory that made nails. He tried to come home every weekend when possible, but after six months, I went out with him. We found an apartment, and we could be a family again.

During this time, we fell away from the church, and we lost sight of what God wanted me to do. Bob had never accepted Christ into his life; he was working two jobs to try to get us out of debt. There was a Vicar at the Lutheran church down the street from our home who would stop in and talk with us as often as he could. He knew Bob was home for lunch between jobs, and he would witness to him. I told Bob that we needed to get back to church and get our children, Bob Jr., and Ronda who was about three, into a Sunday school program.

We went to visit the Lutheran church and attended class with the pastor as our teacher. Bob committed his life to Christ, and he and our children were baptized. This was one of the first miracles God gave us. Bob stopped smoking, drinking, and swearing; he was a totally different man.

We started to teach third-grade Sunday school as a team at the church. As we grew closer to the Lord, our lives became more peaceful and loving. We turned everything over to Him, and as He promised in the Bible, He took care of us.

After our third child, Doug, was born, Bob went to college. After he completed school, the Lord led him to a job where he could use his skills, and he enjoyed it. He finally didn't have to work multiple jobs to make ends meet. The Lord provided us with health and all we needed. Our lives were alive for God.

Things were going fine - we had lived in Ohio for 17 years when we decided to move back to Pennsylvania in 1977. My father passed away while we were living away, so my mother was alone, and her health was failing. Bob's mother was also alone, except for his sister who cared for her.

Everything went well for the next 28 years, other than the normal sicknesses and operations. I retired to take care of my mom when she came to live with us in 1998, before she passed away. Bob's mother was in a nursing home for three years before she passed.

Bob retired in 2003, and we started going to Florida for the winter. We still lived in Pennsylvania for the summer. We were enjoying retirement - until June of 2005.

I got sick.

It started with a bad cough that would not go away. When I finally went to the doctor, he gave me antibiotics for bronchitis. I was getting better, but was tired constantly.

At the time, I was going to Curves four times a week, and Bob and I walked two miles every day. I seemed to be in good health, until this started; I guess we took too much for granted. One day, we walked a mile to our daughter's house, and I could not get back, so she drove me back.

The next symptom appeared the day we picked up the small car we got when we traded in our van. I awoke to a tingling sensation in my hands and feet that wouldn't go away. After we got the car home, I started to go downhill fast. That night, I got this horrific pain in my back, and I lay on the couch for the rest of the night. The next day, as I was coming back from the bathroom, I fell. It was funny, at the time, that I didn't hurt myself; the nerves were starting to go, causing me to lose control of my muscles.

Bob and I tried everything to help my pain. We went to a chiropractor for a treatment, but that didn't help and I continued to get worse.

Bob's Story

I was born in 1939. There were seven children; three girls and four boys. My oldest brother died of pneumonia when he was two years old. My father was a coal miner and farmer. When he was 28 years old, he was in a cave-in at the mines and it broke his back. I think it broke his spirit also, because he could no longer work to support his family. I remember that we moved a lot, as he would try to find work that he could still do. He was limited on many things, because he couldn't lift things or bend over.

When I was six years old, we moved to a farm that had a huge house on it and a large barn and a number of other buildings. I found out later in life that the owner gave my father a chance to take care of the farm and the animals. For doing this, we got to live there free and he paid Dad a small amount of money. It was not enough to pay for all the expenses, so he got some kind of assistance.

My father never owned a car in his life, so when he went anywhere he had to take a bus, or ask a friend to take him, or we had to walk.

We were considered poor, but we didn't know that we were until someone told us. We seemed to have everything we needed and we were happy.

My father became very ill as time went on. He would cough for hours, sometimes. We didn't know what was wrong. He finally passed away at age 41. They said that he died of Black Lung Disease and heart failure.

At the time, my oldest sister was married and lived with her husband in one side of the big house. The owner came to see my mother and told us we had to find another place to live, so my sister and her husband found a place where they could live upstairs and we could live in the downstairs.

I was 10 years old when this took place. The farmer who owned the house told me that if I would work for him on the farm before and after school, he would take that for rent. I also worked full-time in the summer. Then in August, he came to me and gave me a check to buy school clothes, and I was thrilled.

Things were hard for us. My mother was left with five children to take care of and no means to do it. She was totally deaf and had been that way from childhood. She could read our lips to communicate with us children, but she had a hard time understanding strangers.

My next to the oldest sister went into training at the hospital, and she stayed there while doing her job. She trained to be a tray girl who would deliver the meals to the patients. That was one less person my mother had to be really concerned about.

We continued to live there until I was 14 years old, then my sister and her husband found a single house to move into. Their family was growing and they needed more room.

We found a single home that we could rent in a small coal mining town. The rent was cheap, but we had no indoor plumbing and a coal stove in the kitchen and a small heating stove in the living room. There was a sink on the closed-in porch with a hand pump, where we got our water. We made a garden and Mother would can everything she could. This food helped us make out during the long, cold winter months.

I became friends with my future wife's brother, and that was how I met her. I would go down on the weekend to help him do the barn work and we would get done faster so we could go run around. He had a car, so that was how we got around.

On our first date, we went to the prom at her school. We went with her brother and his date, and wouldn't you know it, we were late getting home that night. From then on we started dating regularly and fell in love. We got married and lived with her parents for a while, and I worked for her dad on the farm and at the sawmill.

After moving to Cleveland, Ohio, we decided to take our children to church and Sunday school. This is where the Lord came into my life and changed me into a new person. I knew I loved my wife and children, but after Christ came into my life, I knew what love really was.

When Romayne got sick with GBS, I knew what I had to do and so our story and battle with GBS begins.

As you read the next section titled <u>Journal</u> you will discover that this is a day by day record of Romayne's struggle to get back what GBS has taken away from her.

I, Bob kept a ledger and would write any significant activities for each day. I could not write everything that took place because I didn't have the time to write everything down in detail. There was so much going on everyday that it would have been to difficult to record it all in this ledger. I think that after you read this journal you will discover how difficult Romayne's journey has been.

Journal

I took her to the hospital on Sunday, July 25, 2005 and they tested her and said they could find nothing wrong. They sent her home with pain pills, which didn't do any good.

She was worse that night. I called the doctor, and he said there was nothing he could do for her, so not to bring her back to the hospital. He told me to call our primary care physician (PCP) on Monday morning. I did this, but only got to talk to the nurse. They called in a prescription to the drug store for a stronger painkiller, Oxycodone, but that made her sicker.

I took her for an MRI Monday, and she could barely make it there. They told me to take her to therapy on Tuesday, so I did. She could not walk very well by this time.

The therapist said he didn't know why she was sent there with no diagnosis, but he put heat and electric shock on her back, gave her a walker, and sent her home. The therapist had to help me get her to the car. We had a difficult time getting her in the car. When we got home I had a hard time getting her into the house by myself.

She fell Tuesday afternoon trying to go to the bathroom. By Wednesday, I couldn't get her up by myself.

Our friend, Nancy Schrock came over, and together we couldn't get her up, either. I called 911and had her taken to the hospital.

They still couldn't find anything wrong with her. I was told our doctor asked for a spinal tap and found protein in it. He then called another doctor for a second opinion.

That doctor told him to try to get her to stand. When she couldn't, he diagnosed her as having Guillain-Barre' Syndrome, a disorder in which the body's immune system attacks part of the peripheral nervous system, and admitted her to the ICU in the hospital. I went up to the intensive care unit with her and was helping to put her in bed. The nurse was putting painkiller or something in the IV; as soon as it was in, Romayne had a seizure that lasted a couple minutes. We got her revived and asked her a lot of questions. Just when we thought she was going to be okay, she had another seizure that lasted longer than the first. We finally got her settled down, and they started another IV of medicine and liquids.

The nurse that was working on Romayne told me that I shouldn't have been in there at this time, but she was glad that I was, because I held Romayne down during the seizures and kept her from hurting herself or anyone else. When we finally got Romayne settled down the nurse gave me a hug and said that she will be praying for us. I never saw that nurse again.

She slept most of the night. The doctor sent his assistant up on Thursday; she was there most of the day, checking on Romayne and reviewing her charts. At 5:00 P.M., she told me Romayne was very sick, but they could help her if she went to Westmoreland Hospital, about an hour away. They had to life-flight her Thursday, July 26, at 7:00 P.M.

The staff at Westmoreland started to run their own tests and found heart failure and pneumonia in one of her lungs, which was causing the pain in her back. They began treatment, but she continued to get worse. They put her on Coumadin and Heparin shots to thin the blood because of her heart, but then she developed internal bleeding. The shots were stopped, and she was given seven units of blood and continued on Immunoglobulin, which provides antibodies against certain viral infections. After an ultrasound, they discovered her heart was putting out only 20%, when it should be 60% or higher. They also said they found signs of a mini-stroke on her brain scan.

She had internal bleeding the whole time she was in ICU. The first week, she could not understand what was happening to her, and she continued to lose more muscle control. The next two weeks, she would ask me to help her get out of bed. She didn't know she was paralyzed. I would tell her that if she could sit up, I would help her get out of bed. After a number of times of her asking and trying, she finally realized she was paralyzed. I would move her arms and legs as much as I could, and I would roll her over side to side every two hours. The nurses said I was wasting my time. I said, "All I have is time."

There were prayers for Romayne going on in homes and churches, and even people we didn't know were praying. Some of the nurses were praying for her and said they were praying for me, too.

During her stay in ICU, which was over two weeks, the visiting time was very limited, and this made it hard on me, on our children and grandchildren. Our two sons live in Ohio and would come every weekend as often as they could. The grandchildren would come with them. Our youngest son Doug and his son Connor came to stay a week with me to help me drive back and forth to the hospital, and also gave me a lot of support. Our daughter, Ronda and her son John lived in Berlin and would come to visit as often as they could. She would call every day, sometimes two or three times. Many friends and other family members would be there in the waiting room with me and they came to see her as often as they could. Romayne doesn't remember much of what happened during the first month of her illness. She doesn't remember the helicopter ride to Westmoreland or much about the visitors that she had. Even to this day, four years later she doesn't remember those things.

We were only allowed two people at a time, half-hour intervals, in the morning and the afternoon. This added more stress, especially not knowing what was happening. We were told if she showed any improvement in 14 days, then she had a good chance of recovery. They didn't know how much recovery there would be. The nurses said every time that I was in the room with her, they saw improvements in her vitals, even though she did not know anything that was going on. So they got permission from the doctor for me to come and go as often as I wanted to. I would get to the hospital at 7:00 am and stay until 8:00 pm.

Every day I would help with her feeding, changing positions, and whatever she needed. I continued to pray and told God that He was in control, and that we knew where we would spend Eternity, if it was His will to take her then and give her that peace.

Then on the 15th day, she showed improvement. She opened her eyes and recognized me and smiled. That's the only thing she could move at the time.

God gave us His answer that day, and we began the long, hard journey back. As of today, four years later, we are still going to the gym three times a week and try to walk every day. She still walks with a cane and holds my hand for balance.

She has been such a great witness of her faith and inspiration to others throughout this journey.

After about two weeks, the doctor did another ultrasound of her heart and found it to be normal. He had no explanation for this. I told him and Romayne at the same time that the Lord did it. The doctor agreed and said that was a good explanation. This was another miracle.

Romayne was showing signs of improvement each day. There were little things that I would notice, such as, she seemed to understand more of what was going on around her.

I remember one morning when I arrived at the hospital, she was awake and I was talking to her. I don't know if she understood what I was talking about, but all of a sudden she called out to watch out for all the black bugs on the celling and now they are all over you, too. She said don't let them get on me. I laughed and then she settled down and smiled at me and said I really did see bugs, but I don't see them anymore. After a while we discovered what she was probably seeing. The celling had white blocks with black specks in them. We felt that she was illusionating, because of her medication and we still get a good laugh when we talk about it.

After three weeks in ICU, she was moved to Select Specialty for intensive care plus therapy. I had to get permission from Select Specialty staff and the doctor to continue to keep coming in at 7:00 am and be with her all day. I drove over 60 miles each way. I went every day, and as I was driving I would meditate and pray. The funny part of this was when we would go anywhere, we always would have the radio playing. But I would never turn the radio on, because this was my quiet time with God. At the time, gas was over $3.00 per gallon. This added another burden on us financially, being on a fixed income it put a strain on our budget. We knew that if we had enough faith, God would provide our needs. We were surprised one day when our Sunday School class gave us a cash donation for gas, and then the antique car club that we were members in gave us a cash donation for gas also, this helped a lot. This was another one of God's miracles. God answers prayers, but not always the way we expect him to.

I would help with anything the nurses would let me do. Romayne was still a long way from recovery. They had two Physical Therapists and a Speech Therapist who came in twice a day. The Speech Therapist would help her with swallowing, because she didn't know what to do when trying to eat real food. She could not eat much. They wanted her to have at least 2,000 calories a day. She could never eat that much.

They continued her on Immunoglobulin and restarted the blood thinners, but she developed internal bleeding again, so the blood thinners had to be stopped. They also stopped therapy during this time, just to be safe. She started to improve, and after a week, a stress test came back perfect, and therapy was allowed to resume.

As of September 21, she still had pain and cramps in her stomach and back, and trouble sitting up, but she could also move her arms, fingers, shoulders and parts of her legs very little on her own. I first noticed improvement on the 16th, with more use of her hands and arms, and she sat up for 10 minutes for the first time with three of us holding her. I still did therapy with her every day, and on September 24, I noticed she could move her foot up and down on the floor a very slight amount. She was able to repeat the motion the next day.

During her stay at Specialty, we had a number of setbacks, and they would put therapy on hold. Just as she would seem to be improving, something else would happen. We know that God will not give us more than we can handle, but will give us the hope and faith to face each problem.

She was totally bedfast and had to use bedpans, but without muscle control, it was very difficult for her. I remember when I came in early one morning and she was still on the bedpan. I looked at her chart; she was put on at 3:00 A.M. They forgot about it. Romayne had no feeling at this time because of the nerves. She had a ring the shape of the pan and a number of sores because of this.

I rolled her over from side to side every hour and put salve on the sores. They finally healed. When she was rolled over, you had to put a wedge and pillows under her back so she wouldn't roll back over. At this time, she was dead weight and could not help herself at all.

They had air-controlled air bags on her legs and we had to take them off and on as needed. This was to help with blood clots.

The doctor also ordered a pair of boots, a therapeutic type to help with foot-drop.* We were to put them on for two hours and off for two hours. I did this when I was there, but when I would go home for the night, the staff would forget. There were times they didn't put them on at all, or would forget and leave them on all night. As of today, four years later, she is still struggling with foot-drop.

*(Foot drop or drop foot is a condition where the muscles on the front of the lower leg are greatly weakened. It is

a deficit in turning the ankle and toes upward. Sufferers of drop food generally lose the ability to pull the toes up while the leg is moving forward, and a simple routine like walking becomes a challenge to people with dropped foot syndrome. Foot drop is characterized by steppage gait [drop foot gait]. When the person with foot drop walks, the foot slaps down onto the floor. To balance for the toe drop, the patient must raise the thigh excessively, in such a way that it looks as if the patient is walking upstairs.)

As she progressed in her healing, she continued to have severe pain. The pain was so bad that when we touched her and when we tried to help her with anything during therapy or even when trying to feed her, it would hurt. I couldn't even kiss her unless I barely touched her lips, because she would have so much pain.

The Speech Therapist helped her with words. She was having trouble saying a lot of words properly. She worked with her to teach her to move her lips and tongue to form the words properly.

The Physical Therapist started with trying to get her to move a finger, because she could not move anything. They would take each finger and move it up and down, then they would move her toes and feet up and down. The therapist had her try to touch her fingers to her thumb, but she could not get them closer then about two inches. She worked on this every day. It took months of hard work until she finally touched her forefinger to her thumb. They started with this two times a day, and said I could do the same exercises each hour for a few minutes, but not to overdo it and wear her out. She had continued pain, but she knew she had to endure it so we could help her regain the movement. As therapy progressed, we began bending each knee up to her chest slowly about five times. We tried to increase the amount of times as we would see improvement.

The Therapist suggested we try to sit her up on the edge of the bed, so the three of us got under her shoulders, gently sat her up, then moved her legs off the edge of the bed. We had to continue to hold her because she would fall over. She had no control at this time. As she progressed, the Therapist wanted to try putting her on what they called a standing table, to see if she could put any weight on her legs and feet. They moved the table against the bed and we slid her over on it. She was then strapped onto the table and lifted up slowly until her feet touched the bottom of the table, which had a platform for her to stand on. This was a major undertaking and Romayne suffered a lot during this exercise. She knew she had to do whatever was necessary to get better.

I remember one morning after I arrived at the hospital I found her awake and I could tell that something was bothering her. I asked her if she was alright. She said yes, but I didn't sleep much last night. I asked her why not, did you have a lot of pain? She said yes, but not only that. There was a little china man sitting outside on the window seal all night. Every time I looked out the window, he was there. I thought he was going to fall off. I told the nurses and they said that they could not see anything, (I know what I saw). I laughed at first and then I realized she was serious. This went on for a couple of nights. She kept seeing this china man with his little hat. One day I went over to the window and looked out to see if there was anything that might look like this. I discovered an exhaust pipe with a cover on top that looked like a china man hat on the roof of the building next door. I went back to her bed and laid down on the bed and it kind of looked like what she said that she saw.

The lights at night must have made it look more enhanced. It took me a while to convince her this is what she was seeing. We got a lot of laughs out of this one.

During her stay at Select Specialty, she suffered many instances of blocked bowels and continual bladder infections. This kept her from doing therapy, and we noticed that every time her therapy was interrupted, she would backslide.

She had to go for many tests, and therapy would not continue until they got the results and the doctor's orders to start again.

They decided that it was time to try to sit her up in a wheelchair so she could get used to sitting up. The only way we could move her in and out of bed was by using a sling and a hoist. The first time we got her into the chair, she could only sit 15 minutes. She had so much pain in her back and hips that we had to put her back in bed. They were giving her pain pills every four hours to help ease this. The head nurse came to her one day and told her to try to shift her weight while sitting in the chair, because it wasn't good to keep taking pills and it would help her sit longer. They continued putting her in the chair every day until she could sit for at least two hours at a time. This was a very stressful time for both of us.

During this time, the doctors and nurses came to me and asked how I was holding up through all this. They suggested that I take some kind of medication for stress, but I told them many times that I didn't need anything because I had faith in the Lord, and the Holy Spirit was the only medication that I needed. As I thought about this, I knew that if I took medication, it would not be a very good witness of my faith. So I asked God for continued strength to help me endure this.

We continued therapy, trying to get her to the point that she could be transferred to the Barclay Rehab Center in Westmoreland Community Hospital. The insurance company wanted her to be at a certain level before authorizing the doctors to move her. I was very pleased with the insurance company for keeping me informed on the coverage of all Romayne's medical expenses. They really showed compassion for us as we continued on our journey home.

Physical Therapy said if we could get her using a sliding board to transfer from the bed to a bedside potty chair, and then to a wheelchair, they would probably approve the transfer to the Barclay Center. We worked on this and it took three of us to move her on the sliding board. Eventually we could do it with two people. Romayne still could not help us at all at this time.

After many long days, we got her to the point that they agreed to do an evaluation to see if she would qualify for the program at the Barclay Center.

September 29, 2005, she was transferred to the Barclay Center where she was required to do intensive therapy for an hour, two times a day. She was also required to do things while she was in her room, like squeezing balls, writing words, feeding herself and other things.

OCTOBER 2005

October 2: They got her to feed herself by using a special spoon and fork with a large rubber handle and a special dish. They also had her try to brush her hair. It was hard, but she did really well.

October 3: The Doctor wanted to check her internal bleeding, so they did a scan on her and found the bleeding still present. He said they would keep an eye on this.

She was given a nerve sensor test on the same day. We never received the results back on this test. We asked about it a number of times, but never received an answer. We finally forgot about this test and never did know the results.

At therapy, they showed her how to move the wheel-chair by using her hands and feet. She did all right backwards, but could not go forwards. By October 12th, she was moving a little on her own.

October 17: They wanted to see if she could stand up in the parallel bars. This would give them an idea on how she handled weight bearing on her legs and feet. To do this, one person sat in a chair in front of her and put a sheet around her, then pulled while two other people who were on each side of her lifted her up. We tried a couple of times and finally got her up. She only stood a few seconds until her knees buckled.

October 18: We got her to stand up four different times. The longest time was one minute and 20 seconds. We also tried a different type of sliding board today. One nurse and I could move her fairly easily with it.

October 19: The Doctor ordered a new medication for her and said it should help with tingling and numbness. (After four years, she still has tingling, but is not taking any medicine for it.) She was able to stand three times (five minutes) today with the same help from three people and the sheet wrapped around her.

October 21: They took her over to the kitchen for domestic therapy. They had her open the fridge and get a pitcher of water out and pour herself a glass of water. The therapist asked her what was one of her favorite recipes. She told them homemade fudge. They asked her, if we get the ingredients, will you make us some. Romayne said sure. They brought in all the ingredients and she started. She struggled, but with the therapists and my help she made the fudge. It wasn't perfect, but it turned out pretty good. The nurses and therapists ate it all and said that it was great.

October 23: Our oldest son, Bob Jr. and his wife, Janice, called and said they were coming to see me and wanted to know if we needed anything. Romayne said she sure could eat some KFC chicken, so they brought her a bucket. She only ate one piece and she really enjoyed it.

October 25: There was a big snowstorm when I got out of bed and had to shovel four inches off the driveway before I could get out. I was determined to get to the hospital. The roads were very icy, so when I got to Somerset, I decided to take the turnpike to Donegal, because they usually get these roads cleared first. The turnpike was wet and slick, but I made it to Donegal exit. As I was going down the ramp, I noticed that there were no lights anywhere, so I eased up to the gate and there was a toll collector sitting in the dark. I asked him what happened and he said that all of the lines were down because of the heavy, wet snow and lots of trees were down also.

I was still determined to go on, so I paid him and continued on my way. What a surprise I had in store for me. The roads were covered with slush and there were trees down everywhere. With the Lord's help, I made it to the hospital around 8:30 A.M. With encouragement from Romayne and the nurses, I stayed there and slept in a chair that night.

October 26: I met with the doctor and the therapists, and they wanted to order an electric power wheelchair for Romayne. This was to prepare her for going home or to a skilled nursing home. I convinced them to order a regular wheelchair, because I knew God was going to help her walk again some day. We had her measured and fitted for a special lightweight chair.

October 28: They advised us that they could not keep Romayne there much longer and we should decide if she was going home or to a skilled nursing home.

Romayne and I discussed this. We decided we would try to take her home and I could take care of her. They said they would approve this, but I had to show them that I could do it by doing everything for her like we would be at home. I failed miserably. I could not get her out of bed and onto the potty chair by myself, so Romayne and I both agreed that I would look for a place to take her.

October 29: Romayne was showing some improvement and was working very hard. She started to notice the catheter and it was uncomfortable for her. She had this in from day one, but because of nerve loss, she didn't seem to mind it. They told her they would try taking it out and see what happened, but they had to flush with a large tube. When they did this, she started bleeding in the bladder. They had to take her to run tests to see what happened. They found blood clots in her bladder so they had to run a tube into her bladder and hooked the other end of the hose to some type of pump to suck out the clots and the excess build up of blood. This really hurt her and made her sick. They finally got this taken care of and now they could leave the catheter out. They told her if she voided on her own for the next two days they could leave it out permanently. Therapy was on hold again during this time.

There were many times during our journey when we would get discouraged. She would get some visitors and she would cheer up. We had many visitors during our stay. Pastor John came about once a week. A lot of friends and family came as often as they could, and we had prayers before they left. This, along with our love for God and one another, would lift us up and get us ready for the next challenge.

Her taste buds were all messed up. She always loved her sweets, especially Nancy's homemade peanut butter fudge. One day, Nancy made her some fudge and brought it in for her when she and Wayne and Dorothy and Leo came to visit. Romayne took one little taste and could not finish it. She had lost her taste for sweets of any kind, but four years later, she is back to normal and loves those sweets again.

October 30: A friend and I went to visit a number of skilled nursing centers that had a good reabilation center where she could go to stay. We liked Laurel View and TSU Memorial in Johnstown, but could not decide on any.

As I was going home that night, I had to pass The Patriot skilled nursing home in Somerset, PA. It was as if the Lord spoke to me and said to turn there. I hadn't thought of this place at all. I was almost past, but I decided to turn in and check it out. I know we should never doubt when the Lord speaks to us, and this was one of those times. That became a true blessing for us. The therapy team, nurses' aids, administration and even the kitchen, and maintenance crew became our cheer leading and support group.

NOVEMBER 2005

November 1: We were preparing ourselves to go to The Patriot. Romayne had another bowel blockage. After tests and more scans, they started her on enemas. It took five enemas before they got the blockage removed. Finally she had relief and her bowels began to move regularly

She was very tired and depressed after all of this stress. It was very difficult for both of us, and we felt like Moses and Job and other saints of the Bible. We wondered when God was going to end the suffering, but then we turned to the Scriptures and let the Holy Spirit bring us out of this. We praise and thank God for His presence and for helping us to get as far as we have come.

November 3: The doctor started her on a stool softener called Miralax. She will take this two times a day, as long as she need it to keep her bowels moving. She is still taking Miralax every day and has no problems with the bowel movements. Her bowels seem to be good now. All the x-rays look good, the bladder test was good, a CAT scan on her stomach looks good. We will take her to the Patriot tomorrow, and pray she will get the help she needs.

November 4: We arrived at Patriot Manor at 11:30 am. We got settled in, but they had trouble getting permission to give her medication. They changed the bed from a hand-crank to an electric. Our friend, Nancy stopped in, which really cheered her up. She will begin therapy tomorrow.

November 6: We had a lot of visitors today. It was closer to our home in Berlin, and they didn't have to travel very far, and that made it easier for them to come. The visiting hours are open and visitors can come anytime. This made it a lot better.

She was very tired after this long day, so we decided to stay in her room and order a pizza instead of going to the dinning room. She actually ate two pieces and then rested.

November 7: We found out that the nurses and aids were not trained to use the sliding board for transferring her, so they used the sling and hoist.

She started therapy the next morning and also in the afternoon. She was in therapy about five hours every day, except Saturday, when she only had two hours. Sunday there was no therapy.

She never had such intense therapy as this. We know that is needed for her to get back to normal, if it is God's will. They started with some of the exercises she had done before. They wanted to see if she could bear weight on her legs and feet. They stood her in what they called a standing frame. It took three of us to lift her out of the chair and into the box. They would slide a board behind her butt to hold her in place. She only stood about five minutes and she was exhausted, so we got her out.

November 8: She seemed good today, and was able to stand 15 minutes. She had a good workout - she's getting very good therapy here. They checked her urine test again and found that the antibiotic she is on will not work, so they will try a different one.

November 14: She was very sore in her legs, arms, hands, and back today, but she stood for 15 and 25 minutes in today's rehab sessions She also stacked tubes and hit a balloon. This was good therapy for her.

November 15: Romayne still can't sit long in the wheelchair. It hurts her legs and butt. This is not the chair we ordered, so we hope when she gets the new chair, it will work better for her. She stood up for 18 minutes, then she felt light-headed and said her ears were ringing.

The therapists started to use a new machine on her legs; it shocks her muscles and causes them to contract.

November 18: She stood five or six minutes and got dizzy and ringing ears again. They used the electric shock on both of her legs today.

November 21: We still can't find a seat she can sit in. We are still waiting for the special chair that was ordered for her. We talked to the nurse today about her medications. She takes 100 mg of Azathioprine (immunosuppressant), 75 mg Effexor XR (antidepressant), 60 mg Cymbalta (neuropathic pain reliever), and 75mg Metoprolol (for high blood pressure). She also takes Miralax as needed for constipation and one baby aspirin daily. We called her doctor to get an appointment to discuss with him the possibility of getting her off of some of the medications.

November 22: We tried to stand her up this morning, but she only made it eight minutes, because she got light-headed and had ringing ears again. I called the doctor's office and left a message to check her blood pressure medication, as I think she is taking too much.

November 23: She stood for 20 minutes. We had her lay down and push a big ball against the wall with her feet. We tried to stand her with a walker, and she stood about three seconds, but her knees buckled. They are really trying to get her up and walking.

November 26: She stood on the parallel bars for approximately one minute and 20 minutes in the standing frame. Her appetite is good, but she still gets tired quickly.

November 28: Her feet seemed swollen today. She stood about 30 minutes and did an exercise requiring her to find items in a container of rice. She stood a couple of minutes, with help, on the parallel bars, too. They put a shock pad on her lower legs, trying to get her foot to lift up; it didn't move much, but it may help to get her going. I can put her in bed by just lifting her while she puts her arms around my neck. I don't use the hoist anymore to transfer her. Her feet still seemed swelled up. She lies down and props them up when she can.

November 30: We stood her three times on the bar. She seems okay with it. Nothing new today. She continued doing the exercises that she does every day.

DECEMBER 2005

December 1: I was told not to lift her without using the lift because of safety concerns for me and for her.

The kids were in today – Doug, Marlene, Connor, and our new granddaughter, Katie who was born on October 20, came from Ohio to visit today. *Romayne: I could not hold her in my arms, so they laid her beside me on the bed.*

I really enjoyed the time I got to spend with them. We were going to go out to Ohio to stay with Connor when the time came for the baby to be born. That didn't happen, because I got sick with the GBS. Every time they would come to visit, Connor, who was five years old at the time, would play therapist with me and he would think up all kinds of things for me to try.

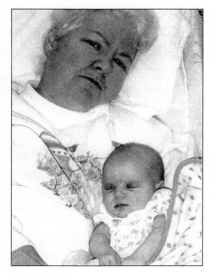

The insurance company called and is concerned about Romayne receiving too much therapy; they are coming in Monday to interview us and are bringing their own therapist along.

Romayne complained about pain today, but she sat up most of the day. She also stood today for about two minutes, with less assistance than yesterday. Therapy said that this was a good sign of progression.

Dear God, as you have revealed Your Love through Your Holy Scriptures, we read in Philippians 4:6 Do not be anxious about anything, but in everything by prayer and petition, with thanksgiving, present your requests to God.

Lord, we need your help more and more each day. We are asking for Your healing touch on her. Relieve her pain and give her strength, courage, and faith to continue on the road to recovery. So many people are praying for Your healing aid, and we thank You for Your love and presence now and forevermore.

December 4: We told the nurse about some of the concerns we have, and she faxed them to the doctor. Romayne still has pain in her hands, legs, feet, back and shoulder. She also has spots on her leg from the shock treatment.

December 5: They put heat on her back. A doctor came in and looked at her leg, but doesn't think it is anything urgent. We talked about her medications, because when I called the pharmacy, they said it was not good for her to be taking one of the drugs, and we should try to get her off of it ASAP. We stood her up on the parallel bars four times, and she stood in the standing frame for 30 minutes. The insurance rep. and therapy persons came in to talk to us, and they were happy with the progress. They told us to stay here as long as we can so it would be easier to bring her home. I dropped the form off at the PCP for a handicapped parking permit.

December 6: She stood up on the parallel bars and took one small step with her right foot; she did this two times, but could not move the left one. This doesn't seem like much, but it was another miracle for her on her journey back.

December 7: She stood up with braces on her knees today on the parallel bars. The first time, she was able to take six steps, and the second time she took four. After that, she was too tired to step anymore. She had a pretty good day.

December 8: She took about 10 steps and stood four times today. We had to hold on to a support belt that was around her waist while she was doing this standing at the parallel bars.

December 9: She had an average day today, and seemed tired. We called the Guillain-Barre' Society, and they will send literature out to us. This is the first time we even thought about doing this. Mark the therapist helped us to do this.

December 10: She did therapy this morning, and seems to be gaining strength. I don't like the swelling in her feet, though.

December 11 (Sunday): a friend from our church called and asked us if he could come in around 2:00pm and bring Diane with him to have a healing service. We agreed, so Diane, Jeff and Pam, Wayne and Nancy, Lori and Pastor came. As we joined hands and prayed, I felt the power of the Holy Spirit fill the room. After the prayers were all over, we all went out in the hall and Diane stayed in and talked with Romayne alone. We could see more improvement almost instantly, but we knew this was going to be a long trip back. With our faith in Christ, we knew we could do it, and whatever God had planned for us in the future, we would find the strength to handle it with the help of the Holy Spirit. We know that because of these prayers and the faith we have, she will recover more quickly.

December 12: She was tired and did not sleep well the night before. She stood okay in the morning and we let her sleep an hour after lunch. When we tried to stand her in the frame, she got light-headed, her ears were ringing, and her eyes could not focus. We sat her down and checked her blood pressure (1 03/68) and her oxygen level (98), but that was after she sat for 10 minutes.

December 13: She slept better and stood 32 minutes in the Standing Frame and 15 minutes on the bars. She still has a lot of pain.

December 14: She took about 12 steps today. We went to see one of the doctors, who took her off the Asthiprine and Exrox. He also thought the marks on her leg were from the electric stimulation, so they discontinued the electric shock treatment. She has to have a nerve test done in March.

December 15: She has another bladder infection. She walked five times and stood in the standing frame for 35 minutes, plus other exercise.

December 16: We tried different exercises today. She walked about 20 steps, but was really tired and did not sleep well.

December 17: She walked about 15 steps with help. She will start the antibiotic for the bladder infection tonight.

December 18: We had Christmas dinner with the kids; Bob, Janice, Ronda, Johnny and Kristi. She handled it pretty good, but complained about pain, though.

December 19: She is feeling better now. She stood up and took a couple steps, after she did her other exercises.

December 20: She did good today, but needs to get some sleep. Her left foot keeps turning when she tries to walk.

December 21: We had her do all the same workout, but we sat her down on a big rubber ball to help work on her balance. She did pretty good with this.

December22: She was tired today and had trouble doing her workout. We let her lie down and take an hour nap. We went back to therapy at 3 pm., but she was really depressed and I had to talk to her.

December 23: She did better today. She stood for 35 minutes, exercised then laid down for an hour and a half. She then walked three times - twice all the way, and the third time only halfway. I went to look at a bigger car so that when she can come home, she will be able to get in and out better.

December 24: She walked two times and stood 35 minutes. She complained about her hands, that they feel worse with the numbness, tingling and pain. Her feet also hurt.

December 25: We went to church on the third floor. She was uncomfortable all day. I laid her down and got her up three or four times. I put her on the bedpan by myself for the first time, too.

December 26: We did some therapy by ourselves today. Also, we talked to a guy in Morgantown named Dave who had Guillain-Barre' Syndrome when he was 59. He is now 71 and said he recovered totally. He will try to stop in and see us, maybe January 7th, but will call first. We had another snowstorm. I could hardly see to get home, and the roads were horrible. But by the grace of God, I made it safely.

December 27: She walked twice, seven steps today. She stands in the frame a lot better now.

December 28: She was tired today and had pain in her legs and ankles, which caused her trouble in standing and walking. We put weights of 2, 3, 4, and 5 lbs. on her legs and had her lift them. She took a nap today. They finally took a urine sample this morning, but forgot to take it to the lab, so she had to do a second this afternoon.

December 29: Romayne was tired today, because she didn't sleep much. She did good in therapy, though. She walked three times after lunch. I went out to Woy's and picked up a van; they suggested I get one to make it easier for her when she goes home. Therapy took her out in the wheelchair and tried to transfer her in and out of the van a couple of times. It went well, so I ordered one, and it should be here by the end of January.

December 30: She slept better. In therapy, she walked seven times in the parallel bars and stood 30 minutes in the frame. She also got her new chair today; it seems to work well for her.

December 3l: They started her on the antibiotic for her urinary tract infection today. She was tired, but walked two times and did her other exercises. I wasn't feeling good, so I left at 7:30 pm. after putting her in bed.

JANUARY 2006

January l: 2006: She had pain in her legs and hands, and rested most of the day. I vibrated her legs and arms twice. She said the new cushion isn't very comfortable.

January 2: We did a little workout this morning and afternoon. She did not sleep well, so she took a couple naps today. She went up to play bingo, too, but didn't win, as usual.

January 3: She walked four times using her old shoes and it seemed to go better. We laid her down on mats and she pulled her knees up to her chest, but not all the way. I'm fighting a cold, so we pray she won't catch it.

January 4: She walked better today. The doctor was in, and I talked to him about her medications. He wanted to start her on a cholesterol medication, but Romayne said no, not at this time. She would like to wait and talk to Dr. Addissie first. He said he would write down that she refused the drug. They also want to monitor her Tylenol intake, so she doesn't overuse it. He said all her blood work was very good, and he wants to x-ray the spot where she had internal bleeding, to make sure it is healed completely.

January 5: She did pretty good today. She can ask for Tylenol, Isopropen, or Motrin as needed. She walked five times in the bars, then we tried the walker again. She walked eight feet twice and one time four feet, while three of us were holding her. When she was trying to walk with the walker, her knees would buckle and she would fall. One of the therapists decided to get down on her knees and move backwards while holding Romayne's knees. This really worked for her. These therapists will try anything to help people to get better.

January 6: She walked two times in the bars and two times in walker. She did a lot of exercises and was tired at the end. She took her last antibiotic for the urinary tract infection today. David called her and will come visit tomorrow. He is from Morgantown and also had GBS.

January 7: Dave and Gloria Sullivan from Morgantown stopped in and gave Romayne a lot of hope and encouragement. Dave said it took him approximately one year to recover from his GBS, but he is very good now.

January 8: She complained of pain in her legs, feet, hands, and back. She took a three-hour nap in the morning, then lay back down after lunch. I laid her down for the night around 7:00 pm., then left for the day.

January 9: She walked 63 feet today! When she walked, we didn't have to hold her much. Praise God! We also got a new mattress and cushion today.

January 10: She had a good day, but did not sleep well. She walked 150 feet total today. She lay down on the mat table almost by herself. Greg tried, with my and Mark's help, to have her get up on her knees and arms and rock back and forth. She then lay down and walked her way across the mat. She took a one-hour nap afterward. Also, they are changing mealtime, starting tomorrow. We don't know how this will affect our therapy time.

January 11: She did okay today - walked 60 feet at one time, then another two times at 20 feet each. They are talking about using the walker in the bedroom. She still complains of pain in her back, and also pain, numbness, and tingling in her legs, feet, and hands.

January 12: She walked down the hall approximately 65 feet, then 40 feet, 45 feet, 20 feet, 30 feet, and 25 feet. We continue to thank God for his blessings upon us each day as we see her recovering.

January 13: She had a good day, but did not sleep well again. She has been urinating a lot at night, sometimes every hour; during the day, she goes maybe three or four times. She walked 260 feet total today. She stood in the bars and bent her knees up and down. They had her use her walker to stand and pivot to get out of bed, get on the toilet, and then get in the wheelchair.

January 14: She was tired and her legs hurt today, so she only walked 40 feet, but she stood in the standing cage and walked in the bars. She stood and bent her knees about five times.

January 15: (Sunday): No therapy today. I vibrated her legs, but she was tired and sore.

January 16: She walked better today. She did 60 knee bends and stood on a pillow and balanced herself while holding onto the parallel bars.

January 17: She walked four times, one time over 100 feet, and did 75 knee bends. She also walked backwards in the bars.

January 18: She was tired but walked four times, about 75 feet each time. She painted her fingernails today for the first time. They had her try to write her name. She didn't do very well.

January 19: She walked really well, about 70 feet, but the walker went too far out in front of her. Her knees buckled and she went down, but we caught her before she hit the floor. It really strained her knees, though. After lunch, she walked five times, but they were short, like 40 feet.

January20: She did a lot of strengthening exercises in the morning, then she walked three times after lunch. The first one was over 100 feet.

January21: She was scheduled for a CAT scan at 8:00 am. They knew that and should have had her ready. I got in at 6:45 am., and she was still in bed. I got her up and dressed, and when they took her for the x-ray, I had to put her on the table and get her off. They tried to put dye in her arm, but both techs couldn't do it. They didn't know what they were doing; they missed the vein, and the dye went in her arm under the skin, making a large lump. They said it would be okay and not to worry about it, but I showed Bryan, the LPN. He did not think much of what happened, he was upset. The lump was still there when I left at 6:30 pm. It took almost two weeks for the lump to go away.

January 23: We had her do wheelchair push-ups. I held her knees, and she could lift her whole butt off the chair. She did 65 of these, and made two long walks. She was really tired at the end of the day.

January 24: Greg wanted to try something new. He stood her up at the bars, then put 3-lb. weights on each leg. He had her lift each one ten times and kick out in front ten times each. She did really well with this. After lunch, she walked approximately 400 feet total. We tried one more exercise in the bars. She was really tired when she got done. Her knees buckled on the last walk, but they caught her.

January 25: She started with 3-lb. leg weights, then 4-1b., 5-1b., 6-1b., and back down, three sets of 15 lifts and kicks each leg. She then stood in the bars and lifted and kicked, then she walked three long walks. She went down through the double door, past the lunch room, but she sure was tired. I left right away because of the snowstorm.

January 26: She had a pretty good day - only walked two times in the afternoon, but did all her exercises in the morning. She helped pull up her pants while holding onto the handrail in the bathroom. She walked in the morning, about 350 feet, then 300 feet, then 200 feet. She did really good at her exercises.

January 27: She did good today, walking and exercise. I talked to the LPN about stopping the Cymbalta, but she said I should call the doctor. Romayne was tired today and took a two-hour nap, but then stayed up until 7:00 pm.

January 28: She tore her milk carton open by herself but could not open it all the way. We soaked her feet, and I vibrated her legs.

January 30: I stood her up, then got the walker and put it in front of her. She then reached out and took hold, and stood. We did this three times. She walked approximately 500 feet - it took 24 minutes to do it. We are trying to get her doing more for herself, so she can go home on February 11.

January 31: She stood at the bars and let go with one hand to scratch her nose, then let go with the other hand to rub her eye. She started to cut back on the Cymbalta to every other night. We had seven pounds on each leg today. She can dress herself pretty well by using the stick with the hook on it.

FEBRUARY 2006

February 1, 2006: We did a lot of transfer exercises. She lifted weights two times and walked to her room twice. The last time, she went into the bathroom. We had her step up on a 4-inch block and back down. She walked through the obstacle course of cones.

February 2: She was tired and sore, I think because she did so much yesterday. We started to walk in the bathroom; as we were almost to the commode, her knees buckled and she went down. We caught her and put her in the chair. Then she stood again, and went to the bathroom. This depressed her, and then the rest of the day did not go very well. She didn't walk as far and had a hard time doing her exercises. We put heat on her knees, and the nurse will put it on again tonight. The doctor called and said to cut her Cymbalta in half until we go home on February 11.

February 3: Two therapists loaded her in the handicapped van and drove her to our home to do an evaluation. They pushed her in the wheelchair down the sidewalk into the house. They tried to see if the wheelchair would fit through all the doors. We'll have to change a few things, but other than that, it went very well. They suggested that we order a shower chair and a walker. We will have to lower the bed because it is too high for her to sit on. I called our friend, Wayne, and he came over and helped me remove the legs from the bed frame. This made it just the right height.

She had trouble getting in the van, but got out okay. She tried the bathroom, bed, and her chair. She went back to therapy and stood and bent her knees one at a time, back and forth. She did all the other exercises, and we had her do small turns with the walker, then sit down in a regular chair. We did this four times.

February 5: She did well today, but she still can't bend her toes back. I put her on the commode by myself and stood her up after she was done; she pulled her pants up by herself. In therapy, she walked in the bars with five pounds on each leg. They started to give her 30 mg of Cymbalta - half what she had been taking. She will take it for a week, then stop altogether.

February 6: Day off of therapy. We soaked her feet and did a few exercises. She had a lot of pain and discomfort in her back, legs, hands, and feet today.

February 7: We got two cakes today - one from Missy and one from the kitchen staff for our 48th anniversary. We got the new van today; we put her in and out four times

- we'll do this twice in the morning and twice in the afternoon all this week. We worked on transfer and turns, plus all the walking and strengthening exercises. We did this so that we would have fewer problems when she comes home.

February 8: I tried to put her in and out of the van six times; it went pretty well. I went to Western PA Sports Medicine for an interview; this is where she will do her outpatient therapy. They have a pool with a treadmill in it and all kinds of other equipment. The interviewer said they had a Guillain-Barre' patient about one or two years ago, and she did well after just six weeks of therapy.

February 9: I bought her a new pair of snow boots today, and now, because they have a small heel, I can get her in and out of the van better. She stood on a rail and walked sideways, up and back; she did really well with it. She also stood at the sink, combed her hair, and washed her hands.

February 10: They gave us a surprise party today in the therapy department. They took a lot of pictures. She will be coming home tomorrow. We pray for God's help in this new step in the healing process.

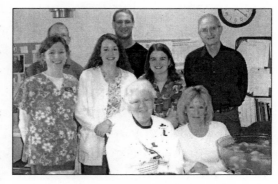

February 11: She came home today. Nancy, Ronda, Carol, Jim, Wayne, Darlene, and Joyce had a surprise welcome home party for her. Everything went well. Nancy made lunch and supper. Kathy Hoffman brought bean soup and pot pie. Leo and Cora came over to help get her in the house and unload the

van. She had a rough night - couldn't sleep, had to go to the bathroom three times, and was restless all night. I got up and helped her get on the potty chair. She still has problems sitting up by herself in bed.

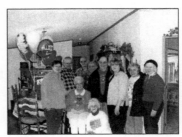

February 12: When we got home from The Patriot, many of our Christian friends set up schedules to bring us lunch and dinner every day as long as we needed it. This really helped us out a lot. Bob wouldn't have had time to cook, and had no experience at it, anyway. Nancy and Wayne came over today and helped walk with her. Leo and Cora came for lunch and helped walk with her again. When we help her walk with the walker, it takes three people to do this, two people to hold onto her arms and one to follow behind with the wheelchair in case she would fall. She also did her normal exercises. The church youth brought chili and stew. We made it through the second night, but she still went to the bathroom three times. She still has a lot of pain and numbness in her legs, feet, and hands. She also still has the pain in her back by her shoulder; this is the same as she had when she went to the emergency room the first time.

February 13: We gave her a shower. Ronda came up and helped - it went pretty well, since we used the tub chair. She still got up three times at night, but I think she slept better. We are going to therapy today at 1:00 pm. for an evaluation. Vicki Rock from the newspaper called to set up an interview to do an article about us.

February 14: We went for the evaluation at Western PA Sports Medicine Rehab Center in Somerset, PA today at 1:00 pm. Dr. Stephen Podratsky said we will give her water and machine workouts, two or three times a week, if she can keep up with doing that much. He said she seemed pretty strong, except her trunk and hamstrings.

February 15: She made deviled eggs today while sitting in the wheelchair. This was good therapy for her fingers and hands.

February 16: She only got up once during the night. Vicki Rock from the *Daily American* was here today to do an interview - they want to put an article in the paper about Romayne. We went to therapy for the first time today at 1:45 pm. She was there for two hours: squeezed the hand machine at 14 lbs.; pedaled the bike five minutes; used the hand bike five minutes, 2-1/2 forward and 2-1/2 backward; lay on a table and used her legs to push up and back; pulled 4-lb. weights with a bar; lay on a table and lifted her legs up and down. They put her in the pool and it took two men to do this. They literally had to lift her down into the pool and back out. While in the pool, she walked on a treadmill, lifted her knees, bent knees back, and walked sideways on the treadmill. He also tried to get her to bend her toes and try to walk on her toes. She walked, not using her hands on the bars, as he balanced her a little from the back.

February 18: We got a call today from a guy in Pittsburgh who had GBS for nine months. He is still walking with a cane, can't work yet, and gets depressed. Romayne told him to trust in the Lord and keep up his therapy.

February 19: We went to church for the first time in seven months, using the wheelchair. It went well. Everyone was happy to see her and hugged her.

February 20: At rehab this afternoon, her feet and legs were still sore after her last workout, but it went well. They continued to add more weights. She could walk better in the pool today. Dr. Podratsky's goal is to have her getting up and standing by herself within six weeks.

February 23: She worked really hard in therapy today. Afterward, we went to Giant Eagle and the local shopping center. When we got home, she was tired and her legs and feet hurt her pretty badly.

February 24-26: The kids were in for a visit. She had a busy week going to the mall and Wal-Mart. This really gave her a boost to see the kids.

February 27: In rehab, they added more machines to bend her knee back and forth. She also walked on a bar sideways with a band tied to her feet.

February 28: Therapy again today. She did the same routine, except the last three programs she went in the pool. Instead, the assigned therapist for the day had her walk up the steps; it did not go well, but he said this was the first try. He wants to try walking down the next time. She has been having more pain in her feet and ankles this last while. Last night, she had pain in her little toe and the one next to it. We hope and pray this is a good sign that the nerves are getting back to normal. She still can't get up herself, but this morning she sat up in bed by herself. She has been walking to the bathroom, just her and I, now for two days.

MARCH 2006

March 2: They increased the weights on her exercises. She gets really tired and her feet hurt after the workout. She tends to get emotional at times, but after she cries, she seems better. She sat up in bed and stood up with her walker. I just stood by in case. She still has good days and bad days.

March 4: I helped her shower today. We tried the shower chair in the tub, but it just didn't seem to sit level. I adjusted it as far as it would go, but it still was not right. I got the idea to put the potty chair without the potty into the walk-in shower in our bathroom. Then I could put the wheelchair beside the door and lift her up to transfer her to the chair in the shower. This worked great, so I returned the tub chair to the place that we bought it.

March 5: We went to Red Lobster to celebrate our anniversary. Her feet hurt, it may be because I was bending them back to stretch her ankles and calf muscles.

March 7: They put her in the pool and used a noodle. She stood on it, walked sideways on it, walked forward on it. They tried a lot of different exercises, like walking on the treadmill and turning quarter turns and walking backwards. She can almost stand herself up from the chair.

March 8: We went to see the doctor about her eye. He couldn't find anything wrong, but said it looked like scar tissue growing on her cornea. But he didn't think that was her problem -she has eyelashes growing towards her eye. He pulled three out and wanted her to see another doctor in one month for a follow-up. He gave us different eye drops to try. He said it might be the GBS causing this.

March 9: Romayne's brother, Jerry, said to try moving the arms of the wheelchair up, so I did, and this morning she stood up on her own. They thought the pneumonia caused the back pain, but she still has some of this. Her legs are weak first thing in the mornings. Her feet hurt really bad again after therapy.

March 13: They had her stand up out of a regular chair with arms, without grabbing hold of anything when she got up. It went pretty well. She has been walking to the bathroom a lot and trying to pull her pants down and up by herself.

March 14: Steve suggested trying a set of ankle supports to help her walk better, and possibly walk with a cane.

March 15: She seemed tired today and was emotional. We need to keep up her spirits. We don't want to have depression problems. I told her to keep trusting in God because He has a plan for her, and in His time, He will give her what He knows she needs, whatever that may be. We will give thanks and go on trusting and believing in Him until we see Him in all His glory.

March 16: The assigned therapist increased weights and moved to Level 8 on the full body machine, and increased time on the bike and arm exercises. She walked 90 seconds on her own, holding onto noodles in the pool. She walked up steps with lots of help, but her feet and legs did not hurt as much as they have been.

March 20: They moved her up another level on the machines and times.

March 21: She walked by herself in the pool for about 30 seconds. Steve had her go down the steps sideways. It went pretty well, but coming out was not so good. They had her step up and down on a 2-inch step. She did okay with this, and she used her walker. Steve wants her to be walking with a cane in two weeks.

March 27: They put her on a new machine that tested the strength of her legs; the right one was 17 and 15, the left 14 and 16. She stepped up on a 2-inch step without her walker, but held Danielle's hand and held on to the rail.

March 28: She walked up and down a 4-inch step today, and got up and down out of a low chair without arms. She walked without the walker. I held one hand, and Steve held the other. She walked in the pool by herself, without holding rails or floats. She did pretty well. She was able to walk down steps and back up a little better when going in and out of the pool.

March 30: She walked about 40 feet with a cane to help her walk. They increased the weights and moved up to Level 9 on the total gym machine. Her feet hurt pretty badly after this workout.

March 3l: We went to the dentist today, and she had two teeth fixed. She said her mouth and face hurt. Wayne and Nancy came over, and we walked her outside. It was 70 degrees. She walked with the walker while two of us helped balance her, the other person pushed the wheel chair behind in case she would fall or get to tired to walk back. We had her walk up the sidewalk and step up on the porch. We sat out and visited for an hour. She woke up only once last night, for the third night in a row. She woke up with a stiff neck this morning.

APRIL 2006

April l: She was upset and cried a lot today. She could not read the devotions. We would always read our devotions every day. We still continue to do our scripture study and devotions and prayer every day.

April 3: They increased her weights on legs to three pounds, and moved the total gym machine up to Level 3 when pulling down with one leg. Steve had her walk with the cane again; she did pretty well. She walked to the room, then back to the gym with the cane, approximately 60 feet. She was really tired after all this.

April 5: Steve suggested that we make an appointment to get a set of leg and foot prostheses. He felt that it would help her with her balance and foot drop. She went to get fitted for leg prostheses for both legs. They said it will take one or two weeks to get them.

April7: We took lunch into the therapy department at The Patriot. We found out that Greg, the one who really helped Romayne, was let go, but he has found another job. We were sad to hear this and that we didn't get to see him.

April 10: We don't need to take the walker to therapy anymore; she uses the cane now. She did the 4-inch step a lot better, and they increased her weights again. Her leg strength increased again today She was really tired afterward.

April 11: She walked by herself in the pool without holding the rails. Matt was there to catch and balance her once in a while. They upped the time on the bike and arms, too. She walks with a cane all the time now at therapy. She went on a 6-inch step; it was tough, but she did it about five times.

April 13: She went up and down one 6-inch step using the handrail and cane. She stepped up, then went forward and back down, with both feet. They increased her weights and time again. Her legs showed improvement in strength, too. She walked in the pool with no rails, on the treadmill. They increased the speed and time, and she turned 360 degrees while walking on the treadmill. She was hurting and tired when she got done. I had to give her Advil for the first time in about a week.

April 18: She walked in the pool for about 20 minutes, not holding on. She stood by herself, also, and lifted 10 pounds on each foot.

April 19: She walked around the house by herself, but I didn't follow her. She did really well. After walking in the pool, she was really tired and could hardly get out of the pool. Her feet really hurt her.

April 22: (Saturday) She had a dizzy spell; I don't know if it was vertigo or not, but she threw up and was sick and dizzy for six hours. I gave her a pill, and she was better Sunday morning.

April 24: She walked in therapy with the walker. She had a pain in her right hip and leg. Steve said her hip was pulled out of the socket, so he put it back in. She says it was better. He wants her to put heat on it and take it easy until tomorrow's therapy session.

April 25: Steve adjusted her upper back, and I have to stretch her leg at least once a day. She was walking with the cane, and Matt wanted her to do it by herself. He did not hold on to her, and her ankle twisted, but I caught her before she fell all the way down.

April 27: Mandi adjusted her upper back again, and she seems to feel better.

April 28: Wayne and Nancy called and wanted to help see if she could walk into the church with the walker. We went up and tried, and she did okay, but was afraid of the ramp. She did great with our help.

April 30: She started walking out to the car with the walker. She walked into church and up three steps to the Sunday school classroom. Wayne, Nancy, and I helped her, but she did most of it alone. They gave her a standing ovation when she walked in.

MAY 2006

May 1: We picked up her braces, but she did not like them. She said they made her feel more like an invalid, but we tried to convince her they would only help her on her way to recovery. She had a lot of pain in her hip, lower back, and leg, and she did not sleep much tonight.

May 2: We went to therapy, and they treated her back and did an ultrasound before sending her home. She still has pain in her hip, leg, and upper back.

May 4: They did electric shock, heat, and an ultrasound on her hip and back. Steve suggested we might see a chiropractor.

May 6: We went to the chiropractor today. He took some x-rays; they show some spurs, and her back has shifted to the right. Also, her back is straight at the bottom, when it should have a curve in it. He treated her with the activator tool, and she said she felt better, but by the time we got home, she was hurting pretty bad. She did not sleep too well again, and says it hurts behind her right knee when she walks.

May 8: She slept better last night. She only did water therapy today. Steve wants to try this for a week to see how it goes.

May 9: She went to therapy, water only again. She felt pretty good, but still hurts. She was on the computer for three hours, then had another vertigo attack and started throwing up. She was sick for five or six hours after that.

May 10: We went to get her leg support adjusted. We also bought new shoes to see if this would help.

May 11: She has been wearing the leg braces and has been walking and sleeping better. She still gets a lot of pain in her shoulder when she sits in any type of chair. Her wheelchair seems to be best for her shoulder. She walked four times around the house, then hurt a little. Then she only got around 1-1/2 times in the evening before her knee hurt.

May 14: She had a lot of pain all night. We hope Sunday, Mother's Day, will be better for her.

May 15: She felt better today and slept well last night. She went to therapy and did the bike for her legs and arms, walked with her cane, and did the Biodex and water exercises. We came home, and she took a short nap and said her knee hurt some.

May 17: We went to see the chiropractor, and he gave her another treatment. He said it looked a lot better. She was sore after the treatment, but will go back in a week. Her pain seems better, praise God. He sure has carried us through so much. It seems we are always asking Him for something, but He will never forsake us or get tired of us asking. Thanks be to God through our Lord and Savior, Jesus Christ! Amen.

May 18: Therapy went well today. Steve wants to order her a cane.

May 22: She walked a lot better today, with less pain. Steve had her do steps again and crossover steps with the rail, then with the cane. She did well, but did not do the pool today.

May 23: She did more exercises today, including side-stepping in the pool and walking without the rails. She walked into the house when we got home, and slept well tonight. She still has pain in her shoulder when she sits too long, and still has some pain in her leg, hip, and knee.

May 24: She walked out to the kitchen with the walker and took her pills by herself.

May 25: She walked around the table while I sat in my comfy chair drinking coffee. Steve made her walk from her wheelchair to the back bike by herself, with only her cane.

May 26: She had another vertigo attack and was sick all day, throwing up and with a neck ache. I called John at the pharmacy and he said it would be okay for her to take her water pill.

May 29: She was a little woozy today, so I gave her a pill and she seemed okay after that. She is walking around by herself now with the walker - going to the bathroom by herself, sitting in her chair by the TV herself. She walked out to the garage while I was waxing the car and talked a while, then walked back in.

May 30: She was sitting in her chair, and she said to me, "Look, my feet are moving!" She continued to move them. Praise God! The movement was very small, but anything was a great leap forward.

May 3l: This will be our first big challenge, going this far from home. We are going to Ohio for Matt's graduation. We got to Bob's around 12 pm.; Romayne had to walk around the house and up four big steps. She did pretty well, though she had to go up and down six times. With our help, she did fine and we had no major issues.

JUNE 2006

June 5: We went to therapy, and she walked with a cane by herself. We followed and had to help catch and balance her. She stood on a wobble board to help her ankles, then she stood on a rubber mat and tried to balance herself; she did not do very well. She then walked with her cane again, but did not do as well as before, but still not too bad.

June 7: She walked into and around the house with the cane we picked up for her to use at home. I held her hand.

June 8: She walked into therapy with the cane and my help. They had her try to stand and balance herself with AFO and without them. She only made it three to seven seconds, but they said that was good. Dorothy brought her a lemon pie for her birthday.

June 13: We went to therapy, but she was sick with vertigo, so we came home. She lay down and took a nap.

June 14: She felt better today. We went shopping, then to Red Lobster. She walked in with her walker and did really well. She started to do exercises today for the vertigo, using a checkerboard. As I move it back and forth, she moves her head and eyes to follow it. We are still doing this every day.

June 15: We went to therapy, but she couldn't do much, because her hip, neck, and back were hurting. Matt, the therapist assigned to Romayne for today gave her a couple things to do on the Biodex, arm bike, and weight pulls, then we left. He didn't charge us for the day.

June 17: (Saturday) I had some errands to run and she said she would like to try staying home by herself for 3-1/2 hours and did really well with it.

June 18: We went to the airport car show today. She cut pies and buns to sell at the car show. We stayed from 8:30 am. to 5:00 pm. When we came home, she was really tired.

June 19: She went down the steps in the garage. I called Cora and Leo to come over and help, but we didn't need them. She walked back up with my help when we got home.

June 20: Steve wants her to try walking with the cane and no AFOs, and use old tennis shoes. She walks with the cane, and I follow her, just holding her waist to keep her balanced.

June 21: Day off from therapy. She got a rash on the right side of her forehead (looks like pimples), and her right eye hurts. We went out to eat and she walked through gravel for the first time.

June 22: Went to therapy. They thought her rash looked like shingles, so they called the doctor to get us an appointment. They wouldn't let her in the pool. When we saw the doctor, he said she indeed did have shingles and gave her medication to take for seven days.

June 24-25: We went to Ohio for Matt's graduation party; she had a rough time with it. We survived and did the best we could under the conditions.

June 26: She woke me up at 5 am. - she had a vertigo attack. I helped the best I could, then got her up at 8:30 am. for a shower. She took her medications and ate a couple bites of yogurt, then started to be sick again. I laid her down and canceled her therapy, but she did go to her eye doctor appointment. He said everything looked okay, but he wants to see her again on July 2.

June 29: Her shingles are pretty well scabbed over now, but still hurt a lot.

June 30: She seemed okay, but Friday night, when we went to go to bed, she was having a lot of pain. We went to the chiropractor again Saturday morning because she has a lot of pain in her back and leg. We played cards later and she felt okay, but started to hurt again that night.

JULY 2006

July 5: Our son, Bob, and his wife, Janice, asked us if we would like to try to go with them to Lancaster, PA, to tour Amish country and go to the Sight And Sound Theater, so we said we would like to try. They felt that with their help, we should do fine, but we had to cancel our trip to Lancaster. She had too much pain in her right leg. We went to the chiropractor this morning, and therapy this afternoon.

July 6: She could not get up out of bed, and she cried. I had to call 91 l, and they took her to the emergency room in Somerset. They took an MRI and back x-rays (I got a copy). We were there for 7-1/2 hours. They gave her morphine, and she slept and felt good as she lay down. As soon as we got up to come home, the pain was just as bad, so they gave her a shot of steroids for inflammation and Hydrocodone pills for the pain.

July 8: I had to take her back to the hospital for her back pain and the pain down her leg. They gave her morphine again, then they wanted to send her home. I told the doctor he needed to find out what was causing the pain, and if he sent her home, then what? He called two other doctors, and they said to admit her. So she was admitted at 1:30 pm. They put her on a painkiller and anti-inflammatory shots in IV. She seemed relaxed when I left at 7 pm.

July 9: They put three patches on her and ordered more x-rays and another MRI. The patches are some sort of medication that is absorbed through the skin; I'm not sure of the name, but it sounded like Lyodone. She still has a lot of pain, and it seems like the only thing that helps her is morphine.

July 10: She had more x-rays, another MRI, and a bone scan done today. She went to therapy and had an evaluation done. He wants to try stretching exercises with her. Dr. Yaros said she might need to get a shot of cortisone in her hip, and Dr. Smith told her she might need an operation on her back. She has a protruding disc on her fifth lumbar vertebra.

July 11: Therapy put heat and electrodes on her back, then did some exercises on her legs. They are still putting patches on every 12 hours - Lidoderm, which contains 700 mg Lidocaine. One of the doctors put a silicone shot in her hip, but it didn't seem to help. Dr. Kates wants to put a shot in her knee. She called me at 9 pm. and said they added Cymbalta, but we decided she won't take this because of all the side effects.

July 13: Kevin, the therapist, tried to put electrodes on her, but when he touched her hip about halfway down, she jumped and started to cry because it hurt so badly. He tried to lay her down, but that only made it worse, so we sat her up. They put electrodes on her and gave her a control box; this is supposed to shock her nerves to fool her brain into ignoring the pain in her back and leg. Dr. Kates put a shot of cortisone in her right knee, then we took her down to the shower room so she could wash her hair and take a hot shower.

July 14: She had a bad morning with lots of pain, but she was better this afternoon. She is going to take Flexadome, a muscle relaxer. We hope this will ease the pain and help her sleep.

July 15: She had a lot of pain at 6 am., and took a morphine shot. She was still not too good at 10 am. She went to therapy, where they put heat on her and she walked two times. They started to wean her off the prednisone, so in seven days she will be off of it altogether.

July 16: She had a bad morning, but then did better the rest of the day. She walked to the bathroom three or four times with the walker. I exercised her legs and feet once, and she walked out in the hall a little ways.

July 17: She got two shots today - one in her hip, and one in her 5th lumbar epidural. She had to lay on her stomach, and it hurt so badly, she cried for 15 minutes. She seemed okay then in the afternoon. I left at 6:30 pm. to go home and mow the lawn.

July 18: She seemed better today, and only took one pain pill early this morning. She stood about 15 minutes at therapy and walked about 50 feet. Dr. Woshner said he will see how it goes the next couple of days, and then either send her home or to a skilled nursing center.

July 19: She called me at home from the hospital around 7:30 am. and said she had a vertigo attack that started around 2 am. She may have to start taking her vertigo medication again every day.

July 20: She was doing well, so Dr. Nicholson sent her home.

July 21: First day home - so far, so good. We are going to do some therapy at home.

July 22: She seemed better today, but she still hurts after a short walk. We decided to quit taking the muscle relaxant because her bowels won't move.

July 23: We went to church on Sunday morning, and while she was setting in the pew with her leg hanging down, this caused her a lot of pain in her hip, so Bob put a couple hymnals under her foot and she said it felt better.

July 24: She was down a little. We exercised and loosened up her legs. We went shopping at Giant Eagle and the local shopping center. She did okay, but was tired when we got done.

July 25: I took her up to the knotting and quilting group that morning, and it seemed to go okay. She went to therapy in the afternoon, and they put her in traction, then did an ultrasound and stem charge, which they want to try three times a week.

July 26: She seemed to be okay today - nothing different. I left her alone for two hours while I sprayed for ants and washed the car.

July 27: We went to therapy. Steve stretched her muscles and then put her in traction and heat for 15 minutes. Then he did the ultrasound and shock treatment. She did the total gym 30 times, then Biodex for three sets of 12 of both legs.

July 28: She had more pain today after therapy yesterday, so she called Steve and took today off. We will try again on Monday.

July 30: She got up and was going to get ready to go to church, but she had bad pains in her back and leg. I gave her a pain pill, the first one in two weeks. It seemed to help a little, but we stayed home.

July 31: (Monday): She was better today, and went to see the doctor. He was happy with her progress, and will make her an appointment with Dr. Oliver Smith to see about surgery. She went to therapy today - they put her on heat and in traction, and did ultrasound and stretch exercises.

AUGUST 2006

August 1: She had some pain today. I took her up to knotting with the girls at church. The nurse called and said we have an appointment with Dr. Smith on August 7. We went to the "Somerset Night Out" with the car club; she did pretty well with it. She didn't sleep too well tonight, probably because of too much exertion.

August 2: We went to therapy, and they stretched her back and legs to try to get all the muscles to loosen up. She had sore calves after she got home.

August 4: We went to therapy and he stretched and did an ultrasound on her back and legs. He had her lay on her stomach on a pillow; it bothered her a little. He wants us to try this at home.

August 7: We went to therapy and did the same things as always; it went okay. We also went to see Dr. Smith. He said he could not see anything wrong, but he wants a myelogram done on August 25 at 7:30 am. He also wants her to continue with therapy with the hope that she will get better. She didn't have to have an operation, this was another miracle. Praise God!

August 8: Went to therapy. Danielle stretched her legs a lot, put heat on, and ultrasound, then Biodex total gym, then went in the pool. She stretched first, then walked forward and backward, four minutes each direction. She used the high-pressure water hose on the front of her leg, and said it felt good.

August 9: We had her lay on the bed and hang her leg over the edge to stretch her muscles. We went out to lunch and she did okay, but she still has pain.

August 10: She walked a little without her AFO, and did okay. She stretched her leg on the bed, and lay on her stomach for 10 minutes. We went to therapy, and they stretched her to loosen the muscles in the pool. She walked eight minutes.

August 11: She had more pain today and couldn't walk as far, but she didn't take a pain pill. She talked with Jean Aubs, a lady who had GBS - she has been struggling with it since she got it in 1999. She is going to the GBS convention. She is still walking with a cane.

August 12-13: She still has pain. Saturday was worse than Sunday. Sunday, we went to church and out to eat at Hoss's, then to the Mountain Playhouse. Romayne hurt, but she enjoyed it the best she could.

August 14: She did a little better today. We went to therapy, and they only stretched her back, did the ultrasound and shock treatment, stretched her right leg, and did the total gym and Biodex machines.

August 15: We went to therapy - stretched, total gym, pool, walked 11 minutes.

August 16: She had a fair day, nothing out of the ordinary.

August 17: Went to therapy - stretched, bike, total gym, pool. She walked 12 minutes. We went to the store and picked up some items; she said her upper shoulder was hurting again now, when it hasn't bothered her for a month. I had to give her two pain pills today.

August 19: She felt kind of woozy most of the day, but we don't know why.

August 20: We went to church and to the Shaffer reunion. She did okay, and walks about four times around the house now. Still using the walker.

August 21: We went to therapy, and she was feeling good. Steve tried vertigo treatment, making her move her head back and forth while he moved the checkerboard back and forth. She got deathly sick from this - dizzy, room spinning, throwing up a lot. She also said her rib on the left side was starting to hurt.

August 22: She did not feel well today, so we canceled therapy and the myelogram scheduled for August 25. She was afraid of getting sick again.

August 23: Went to therapy, even though she was still a little woozy. She got stretched, did both bikes, total gym, arm strengthening, and the pool.

August 24: She was woozy in the morning. In the afternoon, we went to therapy and did the same thing as yesterday. Dr. Steve had her hang her legs over the table, then stretch each leg separately.

August 25: When she got up in the morning she still was a little woozy, so she took it easy that day and she didn't even get on her computer.

August 27: We went to the car club picnic, and it went pretty well. She walked nine times around the house with the walker, but still gets some pain.

August 28: She lay down on her stomach on the bed for 10 minutes, and hung her leg off the bed while lying on her back, five times. She walked 1-1/2 times around the room with the cane. She went to therapy: stretched, both bikes, total gym, push and stretch legs, did both arm exercises, tilt board, Biodex. We will watch and see what happens.

August 29: She went to knotting, then therapy. She did okay, but she only walked 6-1/2 minutes before her leg hurt. She rested for about two minutes, then walked another six minutes.

August 31: Went to therapy: stretched, total gym, bike, pool, and also stretched in the pool, she then walked 14 minutes. We went shopping and then to Dr. Vittone. He finally told her after four visits that the scar on her eye will not get better, and she will have to live with it and continue putting drops in it. We went up and down the steps in the garage because it was raining, and she did okay with it.

SEPTEMBER 2006

September 5: When she got up, she had pain in her left hip. She went to knotting and therapy. At therapy, did stretching, total gym, bike, pool, and walked 14 minutes. She said it only hurt a little, and she was able to go up and down the steps in the garage.

September 7: She is walking better and can lie on her right side to sleep for a short time. She went to therapy and did stretching, bike, total gym, pool, and walked 14 minutes on the treadmill. She had a headache after we went for groceries. She still did not feel well in the evening.

September 8: We went to Nancy's for lunch; Romayne went up the steps okay. We stayed for about four hours, then she got tired. She has been going up and down steps and is doing okay.

September 11: we went to therapy: stretch, bike, total gym, arm pulls, Biodex. Matt, the assigned therapist for the day, had her stand on the wobble board and go forward and back, then side-to-side. He had her walk with the cane two times, up and back. She walked in to bed and stood at the sink to brush her teeth: this was the first time she tried this. She tried to walk in the morning barefoot, but it hurt her feet too much. She has been having a lot of pain in her feet now for about two months. It has been hurting more. We pray this is the nerves growing back.

September 14: Went to therapy: stretched, bike, total gym, pool. He turned on water jets and had her try to stand up and keep her balance. She tried different ways, by spreading her feet apart and together. She also walked on the pool treadmill, 7 mph for two minutes with no hands.

September 17: (Sunday): We went to church and sat where we used to always sit. She walked in with the walker with my help.

September 18: Went to therapy and she did well: stretched, both bikes, total gym, Biodex, arm pulls.

September 19: Went to therapy and did all the land exercises; went in the pool and walked on the treadmill, 1.2 mph for 15 minutes. She stood and balanced with jets blowing on her, and she did well. Steve made a comment that what they were doing before with all the weight lifting and not stretching probably caused the pain in her hip and back and down her leg.

September 21: We went up to church for three hours and cut hams and worked on apple dumplings. We went to therapy: stretched, heating pad, total gym (her leg slipped to the left side; hope she didn't pull anything), bike, wobble board, pool: walked 20 minutes at 1.2 mph. She was very tired when we got home.

September 23: We went to the Whiskey Rebellion car show and helped with registration at 8:30 am., then went to the parade. We helped with dinner at the church, then went home at 7:30 pm. She did really well with it, but got tired of sitting.

September 25: Dr. Steve Podratsky who is in charge of Western Pa. Sports Medicine and Rehabilitation Clinic set us up with an exercise that he said would help her with her vertigo attacks. He called it a 2x2 exercise. The way it works you take a standard checker board, put an **X** in the middle hen as someone stands in front of her while she is sitting down they move the board back and forth horizontally. Romayne concentrates on the X and moves her head back and forth opposite of the way the board is going. When we first started this exercise it made her very sick, but Steve convinced us to keep trying it small amounts at a time. We did it two times a day, about 30 seconds at a time. As she progressed with the exercise we increased the time to 45 seconds. We continued this until she was able to do it for two minutes twice a day. This has really helped her with the vertigo. She has not had an attack for over a year. We continue to do this exercise everyday. She stopped her vertigo medication and has not needed it since.

September 27: We went down to Westmoreland Hospital to visit the staff that took care of Romayne while she was there. We saw most of them, and they were really surprised and happy to see her and how well she was doing. Thanks be to God!

September 28: We do the vertigo exercise two times a day. In therapy, he put the jets on pretty high as she was walking on the treadmill. She had to run a little, then lost her balance and Steve caught her.

September 29: We did our exercises in the morning, like we do each day except Sunday. She wanted to try making dill dip while standing with her walker. She got most of the stuff out by herself, then mixed it up and put it in a container. She then put everything away. It went pretty well. She also walked 15 times around the house.

September 30: (Saturday): We went down to Bedford for apples, and went to Jean Bonnet for lunch. This is the first time she walked in with her walker, and sat on a regular chair. She put both of her socks on by herself.

OCTOBER 2006

October 2: Went to therapy. She walked in with her cane. Steve had her try to walk without the AFO, but it didn't go too well. We increased her vertigo exercise to 35 seconds; she seems okay.

October 3: She was tired when she got up, but I took her to knotting at 9:00 am. This was the first time I didn't give her any Advil or Advil PM.

October 5: Went to therapy and did the vertigo exercise, two times at 45 seconds each. She walked with her cane and in regular shoes. She pumped the bike without her AFOs and walked in the pool 1-7 mph. Danielle turned on the jets twice; she was almost jogging for two minutes each time. She walked 30 minutes. They also stopped the traction program today.

October 6: She got up and I helped her shower, then I got in to shower. When I got out, she had gotten completely dressed by herself, shoes and all. Praise God! We went to Dr. Shaffer (eye doctor). Romayne has to get new glasses; he said her eyes changed a lot to farsighted, and that it may have been caused by the GBS. The left one from scar tissue.

October 7-11: Everything is going well. She is using the walker and cane more and more. She walked against the jets at 1.6 mph and was almost running. We are up to one minute now with the vertigo exercise.

October 12: Matt had her walk backwards and side-to-side (grapevine). He had her walk forward 10 minutes at 1-1/2 mph. She didn't walk that fast backward or side-to-side. He also had her push 65 pounds on the leg-building machine.

October 13: We drove to Johnstown and took back roads. Then we went to Maryland and out to eat. She did okay with all the riding in the car.

October 16: She wore her regular tennis shoes today to therapy, and used the cane with my help. We are going to try to use regular shoes as much as possible. She is not taking vertigo pills at all at this time.

October 17: We went to knotting, then therapy. They tried different things to strengthen her legs. She went in the pool by herself today for the first time.

October 19: She did more land exercises today; she tried standing without AFOs and did well. She got in and out of the pool by herself.

October 23: She is doing more land exercises, trying to get her legs strong. She still cannot stand and balance herself without holding on.

October 24: She went to therapy, and Jackie stretched her legs. It seemed like one stretched more than the other. Romayne said it really hurt. We went to Giant Eagle, and she walked in with her walker, then pushed the buggy through the store. This is the first time we tried this.

October 31: Therapy went well. She stood one minute 36 seconds, then one minute 51 seconds. Steve had her walk over to the bank and then had her climb steps, one foot over the other, two times up and down.

NOVEMBER 2006

November 1: Dorothy called from Florida to tell us someone broke into our mobile home and stole both TVs. They cut the screen on the door and window. There isn't much we can do with this right now. We will have to deal with it later. Leo got someone to repair the screen and window.

November 2: Steve had her lay on her stomach and lift her legs, and had her bend her legs further on the leg press. She will probably be off insurance in about four weeks.

November 4: She went for a blood test to check her sugar and cholesterol levels. I checked her sugar before we went, and it was 102. The nurse called and said the sugar was around 117, and, the cholesterol total was 307 (57 good, 150 bad). She said everything was good and they'd check again in six months.

November 6: In therapy today, she stood for three minutes 21 seconds, three times. She has been going up and down the steps in the garage foot over foot. We try to do it two times a day. She also stands on the bottom step, then steps up and down 10 times with each foot.

November 7: We went to vote, then to knotting. At therapy, she stood and did 'toe, heel, cha cha cha.' Danielle had her do grapevines with the rail, then holding her hands. This did not seem to bother her. She was not as tired today.

November 10: She walked on the treadmill today at home, 1 mph for five minutes. She made fresh pasta salad by herself, except for cooking the noodles.

November 13: She woke up at about 2:30 am. and had to use the bathroom. She got up and on the bedside potty and back off by herself.

November 20: We have been going up and down steps and stepping up and down 10 times each foot. She walked on the treadmill for eight minutes today at 1 mph.

November 21: She walked to the bathroom in her bare feet, then stood up at the sink and brushed her teeth and washed her face. She then walked back and sat down on the bed and dressed herself. She also stood at the kitchen sink to dry dishes, then held onto the sink and walked over to put the silverware away in the drawer. Her ankles still seem pretty weak; we will continue to exercise them. This will probably be her last week at Western PA. Sports Medicine, because the insurance won't pay anymore.

November 23: She did all her exercises, then helped with dinner. She then walked on the treadmill 16 minutes at 1 mph.

We left for Florida November 28 and arrived November 30. We stayed overnight in Orangeburg, SC, then drove on. She handled the trip okay. We were here a week taking short walks outside, then she was able to move around in the house by herself using a cane and holding my arm. Everything went well for a couple weeks, then one Sunday she wanted to try wearing different shoes to church. She walked down the hallway and turned her ankle over. That was about two weeks ago, and she still can't walk very far. We are going to the gym two or three times a week. She does the leg press, arm lifts, leg and thigh press, inner and outer leg press, and she tries to balance. She walks on the treadmill, doing 20 minutes at 1 mph, but she cannot walk on it now because of her injury. She fell down in the living room.

We met a trainer at the gym, and she wants to try working with Romayne in the pool. It will cost us $30 per session, but we prayed about it and agreed to give it a try. We went two times to work out in the pool. Marlyn Black worked with her and showed us what to do. We might get her one more time.

Romayne stands up to dry dishes and cut up salad, and does a lot more each week. She can get in the shower by herself, but I still help her get out.

DECEMBER 2006

December 1: We started to look for a gym that had the equipment and possibly some trainer who could help us to use the machines properly, so she would get the most use out of her workouts. We checked a couple gyms out and decided to go with Kelly Community Center. They had all the equipment and a large pool. They also had staff members on duty, so we could ask them any questions. It was only about 6 miles from our home, so this made it convenient also. We started doing strengthening and stretching exercises, she used rubber band and weights. I would then stretch her legs and then we would have her try to stand up with my help. We started out with 5 repetitions and worked our way up as she got stronger. We did this everyday after breakfast and continue to do this every day even now.

December 2: We finished our normal routine in the morning - breakfast, Bible devotions, stretching and strengthening exercises. (Note: We are still following this routine as close as possible each day.)

We then went to the Kelly Center for our first time to see how it would go. The trainer on duty, Michelle, started her on a machine that worked her arms and legs. She said to do three sets of 15 if she could, but as it got easier, she should increase the amounts.

Then she had her to do leg lifts with weights, then arm pulls with weights. She then had her sit on a table and try to stand up. This would help strengthen the glutes, as she called them. Romayne did all of this with help. She worked out for about an hour.

December 3: We did our routine in the morning, then we went for a walk. She only got about 200 feet up our street and was very tired, so we made it back to the house. We decided to try the pool in the afternoon. She had trouble getting in, but with my holding her hand and her holding onto the rail with the other, we walked down the handi-capped ramp right into the water. She said the water really made it easier for her to move around.

December 5: After doing our routine, we decided to go to the gym at the Kelly Center. She worked out doing her regular program for over an hour. We went out for lunch, then went home. We tried another walk in the afternoon and she made it up to the end of the street, about 500 feet and then back.

December 6: After doing our routine, we went to the pool again. She started to learn to use the water for balance. She would walk forward across the pool, then walk backwards to the other end. She would do stretching and bending exercises, then she would walk side steps over and back. She was very tired after all this. After a hard day like this, she would rest a couple days and only do her regular routine.

December 10: We went back to Kelly Center again today. She did all her normal machines, plus we tried to have her stand facing the wall and let go of the rail to see how much balance she had. She only stood for a couple seconds, then started to fall. I caught her and I got her to stand holding the rail with one hand. This went better, so we will continue doing this exercise along with the others.

December 12: We did our routine in the morning, then went to the pool in the afternoon. She did her walking and stretching exercises, then she tried balancing while holding onto the wall, then she tried letting go. She stood about 20 seconds the first time, then 35 seconds the second time.

The water helps her with her balance. We will continue doing this along with the other exercises.

December 14: We did our routine in the morning, then headed for Kelly Center. She did all her workout and we tried the balancing again. It seemed to go better this time. There have been a number of women who came in when we are there and told her they admired her for working so hard. Romayne told them she could never do it without the help of the Lord. The funny thing is, she encouraged them to keep up their workout routine. She said, "You will feel better after you get done. I admit, I get really tired, but I do feel better. I know when we miss a day or two, I can tell that I really get stiff."

December 16: We did our routine in the morning, then went to the pool. In the afternoon, she did all of her normal exercises and balancing. Then I asked her if she would like to try swimming for the first time. She wasn't sure, but said all right. She wanted me to stay beside her. She tried it and she swam about 20 feet and was really proud of herself. She gets more confident every time she accomplishes anything new.

December 18: We did our normal routine, then went to the Kelly Center. She worked out for over an hour, then we went to do a little shopping. She walked through the stores while pushing the cart. It went pretty well, but she was really tired when we got home.

December 19: We did our normal routine, then went for a walk. She made it over to the next street and back. That was an improvement in her walking. Our friends in the park tell her that they see improvement every time they see us. This gives her encouragement.

December 21: We did the normal routine in the morning, then went to the Kelly Center. She worked out for over an hour and then we went out for lunch. Then we went home and rested for a few hours. She wanted to go for a walk and she walked over two streets and back. We were very happy about that.

December 23: We did our normal routine in the morning and then went to the pool in the afternoon. She did her normal routine in the pool and then tried some swimming. She swam across the pool and rested and swam back. That made her feel good.

December 24: The Kelly Center and the pool will be closed until January 3rd, so we will have to do the exercises that can be done at home and try to walk around the park as much as possible.

JANUARY 2007

January 5: We did our normal routine in the morning and then back to the gym at Kelly Center. We could tell she was not doing the machine exercises for over a week, because she struggled as she worked through her routine.

January 6: We did our routine in the morning and then we decided to go to the gym at the Kelly Center because it was too cool to go to the pool. She did all of her exercises and her balancing went better today. She was even able to do her standing up exercises better today.

January 8: We did our routine in the morning and then went to the pool in the afternoon. She did all her normal exercises and she swam a lot more today. She seems to be getting stronger. She continues to have a lot of pain every time she works out. She said that with the help of the Lord, she is not giving up, so she continues to push herself. Thanks be to God.

January 10: We did our normal routine in the morning, then went to the gym in the afternoon. She did all of her workout, but complained of her toe hurting. I could not see anything wrong, so we assumed it was from all of the workout and the nerves growing back.

January 12: We try to walk farther every time. We walked down Lyndol and around and up Sterling to Dorothy's house, then rested and walked the rest of the way around. This is the most she walked. We decided to take all the curtains down and wash them. She helped me do this and helped hang them back up.

January 13: We went to the pool three more times, then I noticed she had a sore toe that looked ingrown. I squeezed it and the infection came out. I put salve on it and it healed. When we went for a walk one day, she said the big toe on her other foot (left) was hurting bad. We got home and I checked it, and it was ingrown. I could not get the infection to come out. We soaked it with Epsom salts two times a day, and I bought some Outgrow medication at CVS. I called a doctor for an appointment, then it looked better, so I canceled. Then her toe got worse, so I made another appointment for the following week (the earliest I could get). We kept soaking and working with it, and by the next week it was better, so we didn't go to the doctor. She is doing better now, going back to the gym. This set her back about three weeks.

FEBRUARY 2007

February 7: She washed and dried the breakfast dishes by herself.

February 8: She washed and dried the dishes two times today. We went for two walks today, and she seemed to be walking faster. She and Dorothy made "Pigs in a Blanket."

February 12: We went to "Saints Alive" dinner, then when we got home, we walked a complete circle, went up Lyndol, down Esther, and back up Lyndol to home without sitting down to rest.

MARCH 2007

March 2: Her toes started to hurt again. Both are ingrown and infected. I made an appointment with the doctor for March 8. We didn't get to church today because her toes were hurting too much. Bob and Janice were here for a week. I don't think Romayne overdid it, because we used the wheelchair most of the time.

March 8: Went to see the doctor. He said she didn't have ingrown nails, but he thought her shoes were too tight and may have caused this. He cut and removed the edges of the nails. She felt better almost right away. He told her she had neuropathy in her feet. We knew this, because this is a nerve problem from the GBS. We went out and got her new shoes, again. We hope this will help. We will continue soaking and putting salve on for a while. We hope we can get back to the gym and pool next week.

We continued going to the gym and the pool and to Silver Sneakers, which is a program the health insurance companies started as a preventive medicine to help people 65 and over to stay healthy with exercise programs. We went three times every week until we left for PA. We left Florida around the 18th of April 2007.

We got back to Pennsylvania on April 21 2007. She can move around the house by herself pretty well. We walk around the block as often as we can. We joined Silver Sneakers in Pennsylvania, the same program we were doing in Florida, on May 7. We go three times a week. She has been going to knotting too. She sewed a quilt on the sewing machine, using her right foot. She seems to be tired a lot. She helps around the house with the cooking and dishes, she wants to do more and really tries hard to do it, but is still very limited.

She continued regular therapy and exercises at home and at the gym. She still struggles to do little things that we take for granted but for her it's a major undertaking.

We continued going to the gym and the Silver Sneakers program as often as we could throughout the summer. We then left for Florida in November and we continued going to the gym and Silver Sneaker program there. We did a lot of outside walking and this was a blessing. We are very thankful to God that we are able to go to Florida in the winter, otherwise she would be stuck in the house most of the winter months. We returned to Pa. on May 1, 2007.

We are still going to the gym and the Silver Sneakers program three times a week. We are still walking every day, and we do stretch and strengthening exercises every morning. Of course, like everything in life, things come up and we have to break our routine, so we just have to pick up and continue on.

We always enjoyed dancing all our lives. We did square dancing, line dancing, polka, ballroom, jitterbug, and others. We also belonged to an antique car club where we met many great friends. We owned a 1966 Mustang and we would travel around as a group, and many times use this as an outreach to others. After Romayne got sick we had to get rid of the car. Our oldest son took it and is enjoying it very much.

During the whole year of 2008 she continued working hard and going to the gym and Silver Sneakers programs. Thanks be to God she had no major setbacks the rest of the years 2008, and 2009.

GBS has really changed our lives, and we can no longer do these things. But we thank God for all the new accomplishments that we are doing. And so we continue on our new journey and give thanks and praise to Him. Now we concentrate on the things we can do and try not to think about the things we can't do. Our lives are fuller now than they have ever been, (THANKS BE TO GOD).

Summary

God has been good to us. He has blessed us with three loving children, Bob Jr, Ronda, and Doug, six wonderful grandchildren, Tara, Tanya, Matt, John,Connor, Katie, and one great-grandson, Cody, two wonderful daughters-in-law, Janice, Marlene, and a son-in-law, John, who went to be with the Lord in March of 1993, and many other relatives, especially Romayne's sister, Audrey and her family, and her two brothers, Ronald and Jerry who came to see me very often and prayed for me and also many wonderful Christian friends. We had many struggles during our 51 years of marriage, but none were as devastating as this bout with Guillain-Barre' Syndrome. But by the grace of God, we managed to get through them all and we will get through this also.

Romayne has been such an inspiration and witness of her faith throughout this journey. She would and still does encourage others not to give up, but to trust in God and look forward to the life to come, not this worldly life, but especially our Eternal Life.

Romayne still thinks back as much as she can remember about this ordeal. She thinks about and continues praying for all the nurses, nurses' aids, therapists, all the hospital staff and all the doctors who had to put up with her, as she calls it, during her illness. She thanks God for me for standing by her and cheering her up when she gets down, and helping with anything that was needed.

I had to learn to cook, clean, do laundry, and so many other things that I had never done. As I was doing these things, it made me appreciate Romayne for how hard she had worked to raise our family and work a full-time job at the same time.

Romayne will remember specific situations. One that comes to her mind a lot is a situation with a nurses' aid who worked the night shift; this was her permanent shift. She was almost there every night. As you read in the story, Romayne required a lot of help and she knew it was really hard on them. There were times she needed the bed pan every hour, and she had no control over this. She felt bad about being such a burden on everyone. This nurses' aid always seemed to be grouchy with her, no matter how nice Romayne was to her.

So one night, Romayne asked her, "Why don't you like me? You come in here grumping around all the time. The other nurses' aids don't do this."

This aid looked at her and said she didn't realize she was that grumpy. She smiled and gave Romayne a big hug and this started a whole new relationship between them. When she heard Romayne was going home, she came in on her day off to make sure she got a chance to say good-bye to her.

God surely does work in mysterious ways, His wonders to perform.

So in closing, Romayne and I would hope and pray that by us telling our story, we might help someone else, just as we were helped and blessed, to find hope and strength and faith as you will face many trials that will come into your lives. Always remember, the best is yet to come. Through the death and resurrection of our Lord and Savior Jesus Christ, we have a promise of eternal life. God bless you and keep you. Thanks be to God.

Lightning Source UK Ltd.
Milton Keynes UK
15 December 2009

147523UK00001B/1/P